Clinical Ethics

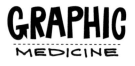

Susan Merrill Squier and Ian Williams, *General Editors*

EDITORIAL COLLECTIVE
MK Czerwiec (GraphicMedicine.org)
Michael J. Green (Penn State College of Medicine)
Kimberly R. Myers (Penn State College of Medicine)
Scott T. Smith (Penn State University)

Books in the Graphic Medicine series are inspired by a growing awareness of the value of comics as an important resource for communicating about a range of issues broadly termed "medical." For healthcare practitioners, patients, families, and caregivers dealing with illness and disability, graphic narrative enlightens complicated or difficult experience. For scholars in literary, cultural, and comics studies, the genre articulates a complex and powerful analysis of illness, medicine, and disability and a rethinking of the boundaries of "health." The series includes original comics from artists and nonartists alike, such as self-reflective "graphic pathographies" or comics used in medical training and education, as well as monographic studies and edited collections from scholars, practitioners, and medical educators.

OTHER TITLES IN THE SERIES:

MK Czerwiec, Ian Williams, Susan Merrill Squier, Michael J. Green, Kimberly R. Myers, and Scott T. Smith, *Graphic Medicine Manifesto*

Ian Williams, *The Bad Doctor: The Troubled Life and Times of Dr. Iwan James*

Peter Dunlap-Shohl, *My Degeneration: A Journey Through Parkinson's*

Aneurin Wright, *Things to Do in a Retirement Home Trailer Park: . . . When You're 29 and Unemployed*

Dana Walrath, *Aliceheimers: Alzheimer's Through the Looking Glass*

Lorenzo Servitje and Sherryl Vint, eds., *The Walking Med: Zombies and the Medical Image*

Henny Beaumont, *Hole in the Heart: Bringing Up Beth*

MK Czerwiec, *Taking Turns: Stories from HIV/AIDS Care Unit 371*

Paula Knight, *The Facts of Life*

Gareth Brookes, *A Thousand Coloured Castles*

Jenell Johnson, ed., *Graphic Reproduction: A Comics Anthology*

Olivier Kugler, *Escaping Wars and Waves: Encounters with Syrian Refugees*

Judith Margolis, *Life Support: Invitation to Prayer*

Ian Williams, *The Lady Doctor*

Sarah Lightman, *The Book of Sarah*

Benjamin Dix and Lindsay Pollock, *Vanni: A Family's Struggle Through the Sri Lankan Conflict*

Ephameron, *Us Two Together*

Scott T. Smith and José Alaniz, eds., *Uncanny Bodies: Superhero Comics and Disability*

MK Czerwiec, ed., *Menopause: A Comic Treatment*

Susan Merrill Squier and Irmela Marei Krüger-Fürhoff, eds., *PathoGraphics: Narrative, Aesthetics, Contention, Community*

Swann Meralli and Deloupy, *Algériennes: The Forgotten Women of the Algerian Revolution*

Aurélien Ducoudray and Jeff Pourquié, *The Third Population*

Abby Hershler, Lesley Hughes, Patricia Nguyen, and Shelley Wall, eds., *Looking at Trauma: A Tool Kit for Clinicians*

Clinical Ethics

A Graphic Medicine Casebook

Kimberly R. Myers

Molly L. Osborne

Charlotte A. Wu

Illustrations by Zoe Schein

The Pennsylvania State University Press
University Park, Pennsylvania

Library of Congress Cataloging-in-Publication Data

Names: Myers, Kimberly R. (Kimberly Rena), 1962– author. | Osborne, Molly L., 1949– author. | Wu, Charlotte A., 1978– author. | Schein, Zoe, 1991– illustrator.
Title: Clinical ethics : a graphic medicine casebook / Kimberly R. Myers, Molly L. Osborne, and Charlotte A. Wu ; illustrations by Zoe Schein.
Other titles: Graphic medicine
Description: University Park, Pennsylvania : The Pennsylvania State University Press, [2022] | Series: Graphic medicine series | Includes bibliographical references.
Summary: "A collection of original comics engaging fundamental issues in medical ethics, including patient autonomy, informed consent, unconscious bias, mandated reporting of suspected abuse, confidentiality, medical mistakes, surrogate decision-making, and futility"—Provided by publisher.
Identifiers: LCCN 2021061074 | ISBN 9780271092812 (hardback ; alk. paper) | ISBN 9780271092829 (paperback : alk. paper)
Subjects: MESH: Ethics, Medical | Graphic Novel
Classification: LCC R724 | NLM WB 17 | DDC 174.2—dc23/eng/20211227
LC record available at https://lccn.loc.gov/2021061074

Printed in the United States of America
Published by The Pennsylvania State University Press,
University Park, PA 16802–1003

The Pennsylvania State University Press is a member of the Association of University Presses.

It is the policy of The Pennsylvania State University Press to use acid-free paper. Publications on uncoated stock satisfy the minimum requirements of American National Standard for Information Sciences—Permanence of Paper for Printed Library Material, ANSI Z39.48–1992.

With gratitude to
Penny Williamson, Sc.D.,
for creating and
holding the circle.

_____

Know that it is possible to leave the circle

with whatever it was that you needed when

you arrived, and that the seeds planted

here can keep growing in the days ahead.

—Center for Courage & Renewal

Contents

Foreword

Michael J. Green

Stories provide a narrative arc and dramatic structure that give meaning to illness. Patients tell their friends and their doctors "when it began" and "what happened next." Doctors tell stories when they talk among themselves, when they present formally at rounds, and when they write reports for peer-reviewed publication (Shapiro, Bezzubova, and Koons). Throughout my twenty-five-plus years of teaching clinical ethics to medical students, I have witnessed positive responses from students to the stories in the clinical cases they study, as students find stories more accessible and engaging than abstract philosophical discussions of principles and theory. Because stories are so appealing, the case presentation format is used by healthcare providers to share clinical information and has been adopted by ethicists to present and disseminate ethics cases as well.

Even so, text-based ethics case presentations have limitations. Modeled after the medical case presentation, ethics cases generally adopt the manner of a dispassionate observer, using a style meant to signify objectivity by supplying reliable raw data on which subsequent analysis is based. However, as humanities scholar Todd Chambers argues in his book *The Fiction of Bioethics*, the problem with this approach is that case presentations are anything but objective; rather, they are constructed narratives that inevitably reflect the authors' biases, moral point of view, and framing under the guise of "real life." Chambers describes how the typical construction of ethics cases appropriates the style and traits of the medical case, including the ample use of passive voice and clinical sterility. In doing so, ethics cases "do not tell the patient's story, nor do they tell . . . the ethicist's story; instead, they tell the physician's story" (25).

As such, ethics case presentations function like a wolf in sheep's clothing: they provide a veneer of objectivity, leaving readers with the impression that the cases are written with impartiality and omniscience. But this belies reality. Without a transparent accounting of who is writing the case and what the biases are, it is difficult for readers to fully appreciate the complexity of the stories being considered.

So, what does this have to do with a book that uses comics to tell stories from the arena of medical ethics? As colorfully described by comics artist Steven Keewatin Sanderson, at first blush comics and medicine seem like mustard and pudding—they simply don't belong together. But, upon deeper exploration, it turns out that comics offer a way of communicating that is different from, and sometimes better than, standard text-only case presentations. And for the particular task of exploring the ethical dimensions of medical encounters, comics offer a new way to engage readers in the complexity of ethical problems.

Unlike standard, ostensibly "neutral" case presentations where the author's identity and voice are typically opaque, "comics are unabashedly subjective" (Kuttner et al. 11). The comics artist is at once producer, director, writer, editor, and actor, and her decisions influence every aspect of the reader's experience and understanding of the case. The choices for which the comics artist is responsible are seemingly limitless: *Whose point of view is portrayed? Where does the scene start? When does it end? What is included in the story and what is excluded? What is shown visually and what is told verbally? How do the words relate to the images? What happens between the comic panels, and how do we know that? How is time portrayed? What is the hierarchal relationship between characters?* The answer to each of these questions signals a series of choices, and the result is a distinctive point of view that manifests social, cultural, and economic norms and expectations, which has profound implications for how the case is understood.

Some scholars have described what the comics medium "affords"—that is, what the medium offers and promises as a result of its properties (Kuttner et al.). Comics are typically understood to be visual stories, usually told through the juxtaposition of images and text, occurring in sequence. They are lauded for their ability to communicate vast amounts of information economically, using less space and requiring less time from the reader. Comics are generally easy to access, digest, and comprehend, and are particularly effective at communicating emotions, context, and time. Increasingly, comics are used in educational settings for teaching diverse learners and topics, including cultural studies, science, law, and even medicine (Czerwiec et al.). Though comics have made a few forays into the field of medical ethics (Elghafri; Olmsted and Green), this is a promising new area of opportunity.

That said, does the world need another ethics casebook, particularly one that takes the form of a comic? After all, comics can carry cultural baggage, such as their use of stereotypes to categorize people into archetypes and their historical connection to superheroes and kids. Yes! Because comics are so much more than this, and they have the capacity to help readers think differently about ethical conundrums through their use of visual metaphors and clever narrative structure. Consider the following ways that comics can be an especially effective tool for communicating the complexity of ethical issues in clinical medicine.

First, reading comics can convey more meaning than reading text alone, as it involves interrogating images as well as words. It has been said that a picture is worth a thousand words, and for good reason. Images contain information that is difficult to glean from words alone, such as body language, facial expression, and contradictions between what is said and what is felt. All of this information can be relevant for understanding the origins of an ethical dilemma and the biases and barriers to resolving it.

Second, comics can foster empathy. As noted by physician and comics artist Ian Williams, reading a comic can be a portal into an individual's experience, insofar as it "creat[es] empathic bonds between the author and the reader" (354). This empathic connection between author and reader is in marked contrast to the typical ethics case presentation, where the author's footprint is so invisible it's easy to forget that someone actually constructed the presentation and made choices about what, when, and how to convey the material. In comics, we have insight into the inner lives of characters in ways that help the reader imagine what someone else is experiencing. Prominent comics scholar and artist Scott McCloud surmises that one reason readers relate to the cartoonish characters found in comics is that these drawings are abstractions that focus on essential meanings. By simplifying human features in a cartoony way, an image becomes more universal and hence applies to more people (fig. 1). Using the example of a face, McCloud notes that the less specific the image, the more the readers are able to recognize and see themselves (36).

THUS, WHEN YOU LOOK AT A PHOTO OR REALISTIC DRAWING OF A FACE--
--YOU SEE IT AS THE FACE OF ANOTHER.
BUT WHEN YOU ENTER THE WORLD OF THE CARTOON--
--YOU SEE YOURSELF.

Fig. 1
From Scott McCloud, *Understanding Comics: The Invisible Art* (New York: Harper Perennial, 1994).

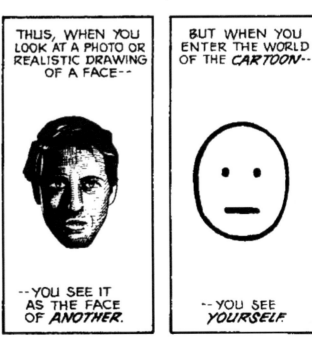

Third, reading a comic requires active involvement in the construction and completion of the story. Text-based cases tend to be passive: the presenter reports a series of events, the reader takes it in, and then discussion and analysis follow. Comics work differently; by their very nature, comics cannot show everything, so the reader must fill in missing information to complete the story. Each comics panel represents a moment in time, and the next panel represents a different moment that might occur seconds, minutes, or years later, or even in the past. Sometimes the moment is a memory or a dream, and sometimes it is the same moment told from someone else's point of view. In any event, the reader must infer what (if anything) happened in the space between the panels (or "gutter," as it is known), and this requires the active involvement of the reader to finish the story. So in this way, the reader is co-constructing the narrative, and the illusion of authorial objectivity is exposed—which differentiates comics-based case presentations from standard versions.

By way of example, let's compare a standard text-based ethics case presentation with a comics version. Perusing the half dozen or so ethics casebooks on my bookshelves, I notice a familiar pattern in the standard cases: an anonymous author describes a medical situation that caused someone (typically the healthcare provider) to experience distress. This "case" is described as "real" and the clinician is often uncertain or conflicted about what is the right thing to do. Consider the following:

> Mr. S. P., a 55-year-old teacher, has experienced chest pains and several fainting spells during the past 3 months. He reluctantly visits a physician at his wife's urging. He is very nervous and anxious and says to the physician at the beginning of the interview that he abhors doctors and hospitals. On physical examination, he has classic signs of tight aortic stenosis, confirmed by echocardiogram. The physician wants to recommend cardiac catheterization and probably cardiac surgery. However, given his impression of this patient, the physician is worried that full disclosure of the risks of catheterization would lead the patient to refuse the procedure. (Jonsen et al. 68)

Fundamentally, the case is about whether and how to elicit meaningful informed consent for a clinical procedure. Though the case is presented from the physician's point of view, we aren't provided any information about the doctor himself, his relevant experiences, biases, or competing responsibilities. Nor do we hear the patient's voice, only the doctor's recollection of a prior conversation and his interpretation of how the patient might respond. The case raises some questions about informed consent and its challenges but does very little to provide insight into the underlying reasons for these problems.

Contrast this to a comics-based case on a similar topic. In *The Swan* comic in this book, the medical team is shown visiting a hospitalized patient in the intensive care unit. Seen from the vantage point of the attending physician, a trainee presents the case of a patient with heart failure. The medical team believes they need more information to properly treat the patient, and the attending physician declares that a pulmonary artery catheter (or "swan," as it is colloquially known) could be useful. He approaches the patient with the intent of getting him to sign the consent form, and in doing so, casually mentions (while texting on his phone) that it's so "we can put the swan in your chest."

Several aspects of this largely visual story differentiate it from the standard approach. First and most obviously, the story is multimodal. That is, it communicates using both text and images, with each "mode" contributing something essential to the meaning of the story. The words themselves provide an incomplete picture: "Hello, Mr. and Mrs. Porter. I need you to sign this consent form. Then we can put the swan in your chest." The visual elements offer something different—a discordant message showing a distracted doctor tapping on his phone and avoiding eye contact. When juxtaposed with the words, we understand that the doctor is disengaged and failing to pay close attention to the patient and his concerns, which results in failed communication and dramatic misunderstanding on the part of the patient and his wife.

Second, the comic provides competing versions of the same story, sometimes even simultaneously. Rather than privilege the doctor's voice as the single arbiter of truth, it reveals the complexity of communication by juxtaposing the patient's point of view. Initially, the reader sees only what the doctor would see as he holds a phone in one hand and extends a consent form in the other. But then we view the patient's radically different perspective, presented via a thought balloon where he imagines what the doctor's words would mean for him. This shift in perspective implicitly raises questions about whose voice matters in the story and which perspective represents "the truth" with regard to the patient's experience.

Third, the comic manifests a point of view. Rather than presenting the story in the typical dispassionate manner of a standard case presentation, it proudly wears its biases. The reader can immediately see and experience how and why informed consent was unsuccessful, as reflected by the authors' use of visual imagery, shifting perspective, and eventual mea culpa of the doctor. The comic doesn't simply tell readers about the elements of informed consent; it shows them why this matters, what it means, and how to elicit it successfully. By shifting the point of view from that of the doctor (What task do I need to perform?) to that of the patient (What do I need to understand?), the comic engages the reader in the lived experience of decision-making during critical illness.

For all these reasons, using comics to present clinical ethics cases is both informative and radical. The medium can help readers understand the complexity of human experiences that can lead to ethical dilemmas, and it offers a more complete and robust way to show the human aspects of clinical stories than is often found in formulaic, text-based case presentations. The comics that follow are innovative not only for their creative mode of presentation but also for their effect: they invite readers to engage with ethical dilemmas both cognitively and emotionally, asking readers to see *and* feel the stories. These visually engaging original source materials make a welcome addition to any bookshelf or library and can be used by students, teachers, and anyone else who wishes to explore, discuss, and debate ethical issues in medicine. So bring on the comics!

References

Chambers, Tod. *The Fiction of Bioethics: Cases as Literary Texts.* Routledge, 1999.

Czerwiec, M. K., Ian Williams, Susan Squier, Michael J. Green, Kimberly R. Myers, and Scott T. Smith. *Graphic Medicine Manifesto.* Penn State University Press, 2015.

Elghafri, Amani A. "Integrating Comics into Medical Ethics Education: Medical and Physician Assistant Students' Perspectives." Master's thesis, Harvard Medical School, 2017.

Jonsen, Albert R., Mark Siegler, and William J. Winslade. *Clinical Ethics: A Practical Approach to Ethical Decisions in Clinical Medicine.* 6th ed., McGraw-Hill, 2006.

Kuttner, Paul J., Marcus B. Weaver-Hightower, and Nick Sousanis. "Comics-Based Research: The Affordances of Comics for Research Across Disciplines." *Qualitative Research*, vol. 21, no. 2, June 5, 2020, doi:10.1177/1468794120918845.

McCloud, Scott. *Understanding Comics: The Invisible Art.* Harper Perennial, 1994.

Olmsted, Taylor, and Michael J. Green. "Comics and the Ethics of Representation in Health Care." *AMA Journal of Ethics*, vol. 20, no. 2, 2018, pp. 130–33.

Sanderson, Steven Keewatin. Keynote address. Comics and Medicine 6th International Conference: Spaces of Care, July 17, 2015, Culver Arts Center, Riverside, CA.

Shapiro, Johanna, Elena Bezzubova, and Ronald Koons. "Medical Students Learn to Tell Stories About Their Patients and Themselves." *Virtual Mentor*, vol. 13, no. 7, 2011, pp. 466–70.

Williams, Ian. "Autography as Auto-Therapy: Psychic Pain and the Graphic Memoir." *Journal of Medical Humanities*, vol. 32, no. 4, 2011, pp. 353–66.

Acknowledgments

We are deeply grateful to the following individuals for allowing us to render their stories—either personal or created as ethics cases—in comic form: Dennis L. Gingrich, M.D., for *Battered Trust*; Benjamin H. Levi, M.D., Ph.D., for *Sneaking Suspicion*; Laura T. Blanchard, M.D., for personal details in *Sneaking Suspicion*; and Dennis H. Novack, M.D., and Janet Fleetwood, Ph.D., for *Charting Courses*.

We also offer warm thanks to our ethicist colleagues in the Department of Humanities at Penn State College of Medicine—Michael J. Green, M.D.; Benjamin H. Levi, M.D., Ph.D.; and Rebecca Volpe, Ph.D.—whose expert framing of ethical issues in their Medical Ethics and Professionalism course is reflected in the brief essays that accompany each comic. Your disciplinary expertise and pedagogical creativity are foundational to this work.

This book would not exist without generous grants from the Doctors Kienle Center for Humanistic Medicine (Penn State College of Medicine) and the Oregon Health and Science University that funded the majority of Zoe's drawing. Thanks for your support!

We would like to acknowledge the Doctors Kienle Center for Humanistic Medicine further for sponsoring Molly and Charlotte as Kienle visiting scholars, enabling them to come to Penn State College of Medicine in 2017 to work with Kimberly in order to move this project forward. It was during this time that we connected with Zoe.

Our respective institutions have facilitated our work in important ways. Molly gives special thanks to the VA Portland Health Care System for supporting the Integrated Ethics Program and giving her the opportunity to share published vignettes in teaching and at ethics conferences. Charlotte thanks the Department of General Internal Medicine, Boston University School of Medicine, and Boston Medical Center for supporting the academic time she dedicated to this project. And Kimberly thanks the Department of Humanities, Penn State College of Medicine, and the Pennsylvania State University for providing a sabbatical to complete this book. Special thanks to Michael Green for his support as interim department chair and for helpful feedback on the penultimate drafts of comics and essays.

We're grateful to the editorial collective of the Penn State University Press Graphic Medicine series for believing in our project and to assistant director and editor in chief at PSUP, Kendra Boileau, for her guidance through each phase of this work.

Jim Thomas, retired dean of fine arts, gifted us with his time and sharp editorial skills by reading the manuscript and offering excellent insights from the perspective of a lay reader, the core of our intended audience. Thanks, Jim!

Finally, we thank Penny Williamson, Ph.D., for convening and nurturing the "Courage to Lead" community on Cape Cod, where Charlotte, Molly, and Kimberly first met and where this project was born.

Introduction

This book is an exploration of common ethical dilemmas that occur in the context of clinical medicine. Such quandaries emerge in interactions among key stakeholders, including patients, their families, and various members of healthcare provider teams. Clinical ethics involves stories of patients, known as "cases," and each of the eight original comics here presents a case that focuses on a particular topic, such as *unconscious bias*, *confidentiality*, and *mandated reporting of suspected abuse*. It is important to keep in mind, however, that discussion of one ethical concept often leads to discussion of others, as ethical concepts and conundrums frequently overlap. For instance, one cannot talk about *informed consent* without also considering patient *autonomy*. For this reason, our collection of graphic stories is highly intertextual: the comics "speak" to one another. Reflecting on one case may shift a person's perception of the others.

The comics included here are based on real cases, though we have modified some details in order to maintain confidentiality and keep the focus on key ethical topics. In some instances, this process included changing the resolution of the story. Additionally, we chose to withhold a decision or final outcome in several comics to provoke rigorous discussion of what happened, what might have happened, and what factors could influence potential outcomes. Because most ethical dilemmas are messy, complex, and challenging, the comics presented here do not have "tidy resolutions"; they are designed to illustrate the stickiness of real-life scenarios.

To provide further information about the ethical issue at hand, we include a brief discussion after each comic (e.g., a short essay on medical mistakes and truth-telling after *Battered Trust*). The essays incorporate illustrative details and methods of conceptual "framing" utilized by our ethicist colleagues at Penn State College of Medicine—Michael Green, Benjamin Levi, and Rebecca Volpe—in their Medical Ethics and Professionalism course for second-year medical students and in their ethics rounds.

We provide questions for further reflection, too. These questions are intended to invite deeper consideration of the ethical issues addressed in the comic and also to point readers to ideas and details they might not have considered while reading: subtleties in the comic's images and words, nuances of the ethical deliberations, and broader personal and societal implications raised by the story.

After each comic we also offer a short list of related readings for those who want to investigate topics more broadly. These pieces are chosen to appeal to a wide range of readers; most are story-based and many appear in *The Social Medicine Reader* (SMR), edited by Gail Henderson and colleagues. The *SMR* anthology is an excellent resource for anyone interested in biomedical ethics and other issues related to humanities and social sciences in healthcare, so we provide bibliographic information for the readings as they appear in that book for the convenience of our readers who might want to add it to their libraries.

Finally, basic to any understanding of biomedical ethics is familiarity with four fundamental moral principles: beneficence, nonmaleficence, autonomy, and justice. Collectively, these ideals are known as "principlism," which is arguably the most widely known and consistently utilized ethics framework. (Other conceptual models include feminist ethics, narrative ethics, deontology, and casuistry.) Theoretically, every dilemma in medical ethics can be interpreted and deliberated using these primary principles.

Beneficence means doing good—acting in a patient's best interests and consciously promoting positive outcomes. To act with beneficence, a healthcare provider must assess the respective benefits and burdens (or risks) of a situation and choose interventions that maximize the former while minimizing the latter.

Nonmaleficence is the principle of avoiding harm. Before beginning medical practice, physicians take the Hippocratic oath, which includes a commitment to "first, do no harm." Nonmaleficence sometimes emerges as a decision to refrain from a particular treatment that could potentially be more harmful than beneficial.

Autonomy is the idea that persons have the right to self-rule, to make decisions for themselves and control their own lives. In order to exercise autonomy, a person must be free from controlling influences, including other people who would withhold or selectively share information, and any other covert factors that might interfere with the ability to make independent decisions. To act autonomously, a person must understand a situation fully and be able to communicate how she wants to respond to it.

Justice concerns treating people with equality, fairness, and consistency. Discussions of different types of justice often emerge in times of shortage: Who gets scarce resources and who doesn't? Are like persons treated similarly (egalitarian justice), or will only those most likely to survive receive medical care (utilitarian justice)?

While on the surface these principles might seem distinct, straightforward, and even simple, they in fact almost always intersect and overlap and are frequently at odds with one another in an ethical debate. Take, for instance, the issue of vaccination. As this book goes to press early in 2021, the world is in the grip of COVID-19. This coronavirus is currently responsible for the deaths of more than 4,000 U.S. citizens—and some 15,500 individuals worldwide—*every day*. Two vaccines have recently been granted Emergency Use Authorization, and the demand for them is high; many people view vaccination as the best way to avoid contagion and death. Not incidentally, vaccination is also seen as the most promising way to return to some semblance of normal life, which is increasingly urgent after almost a year in various forms of lockdown. In this context, providing the vaccination is viewed as an act of benevolence. But what about instances in which a patient is both at very high risk for contracting the disease and also has a history of allergic reactions to vaccinations for other diseases? Here, the healthcare provider must carefully weigh beneficence and nonmaleficence to determine her recommendation to the patient. And the (adult) patient must then decide for herself the degree to which she is willing to risk unpleasant or even life-threatening side effects in hopes of protecting herself from the ravages of the disease.

Few people question the rightness of autonomy as it impacts only the patient. But what about when the impact of a personal decision has ramifications for others? Such is the case with so-called anti-vaxxers, who believe it's too soon to know long-term effects of these new vaccinations and therefore refuse to vaccinate themselves and their children. How can one ethically arbitrate between anti-vaxxer parents who fear and refuse vaccinations and parents who, for instance, argue that their children have a right to attend school without increased risk of exposure to infection? This nexus of autonomy, nonmaleficence, and beneficence is particularly complex, as it moves beyond the bounds of one-on-one clinical medicine and demands response on a larger societal, and often legal, scale.

Complicating matters further, demand for vaccines currently far outweighs supply. Who should receive this potentially lifesaving treatment—and when? On what basis are these decisions made? While the federal Centers for Disease Control and Prevention (CDC) in the United States has issued guidelines, individual states are left to determine ethically just processes. Does providing online registration enhance fair distribution of this valuable resource, or does it disadvantage already disadvantaged populations like the poor, who might not be able to afford internet service, and the elderly, who might not understand or utilize such technology?

Ideally, each of the four fundamental principles carries the same weight, but in practice some principles are more highly valued than others. For example, individual autonomy tends to predominate in the twenty-first-century United States. That said, individual autonomy does not necessarily predominate in places with different access to resources, or where the culture places a high value on family- or community-based decision-making.

These issues are thorny. We hope that the comics we've created spark insights and conversations about areas of medicine that can be controversial and, more, that they illuminate our shared humanity. We're glad you have chosen to join us.

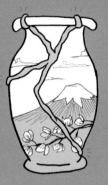

Chapter 1

Autonomy

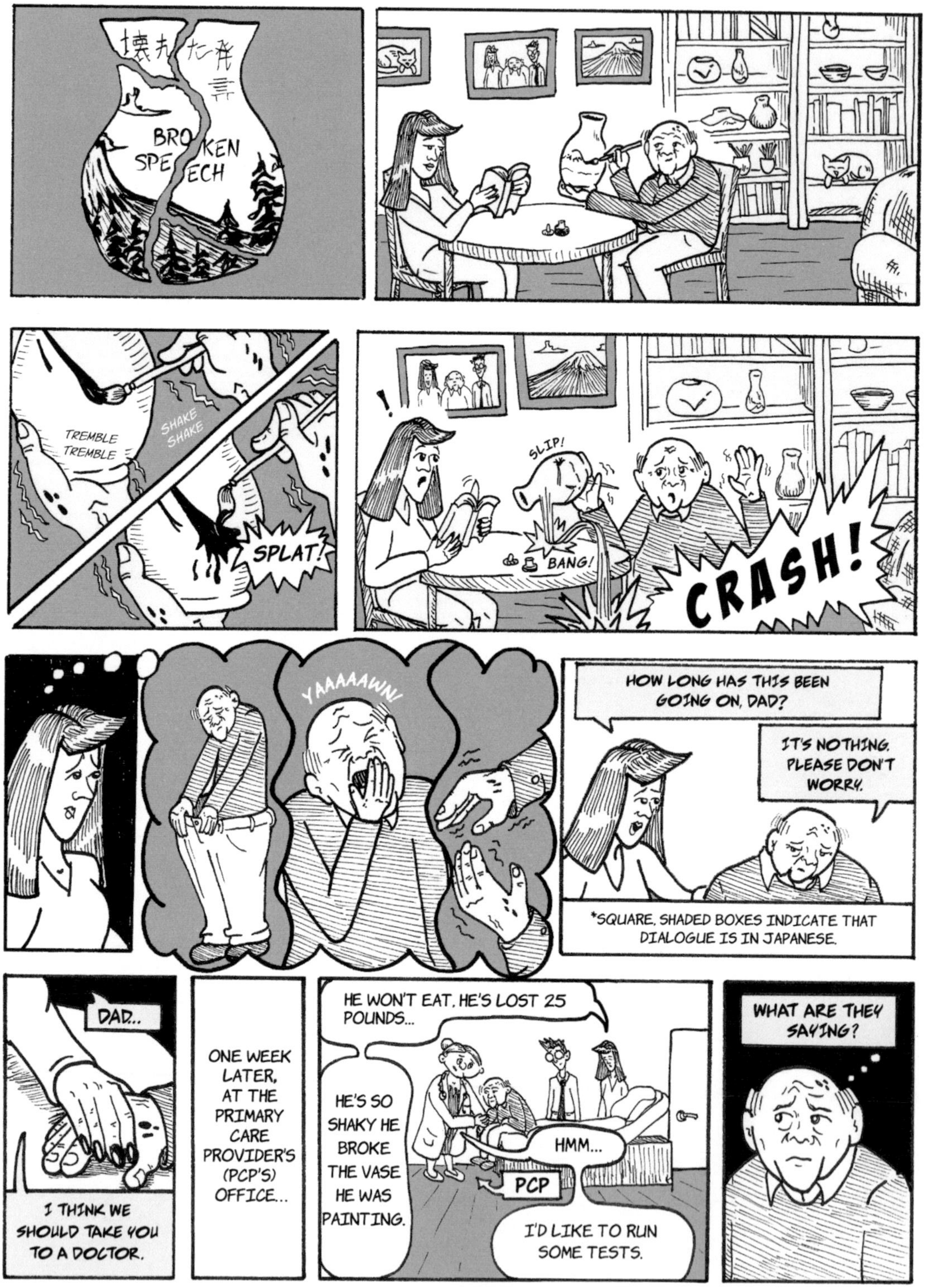
壊れた発言
BROKEN SPEECH
TREMBLE TREMBLE
SHAKE SHAKE
SPLAT!
!
SLIP!
BANG!
CRASH!
YAAAAAWN!
HOW LONG HAS THIS BEEN GOING ON, DAD?
IT'S NOTHING. PLEASE DON'T WORRY.
*SQUARE, SHADED BOXES INDICATE THAT DIALOGUE IS IN JAPANESE.
DAD...
I THINK WE SHOULD TAKE YOU TO A DOCTOR.
ONE WEEK LATER, AT THE PRIMARY CARE PROVIDER'S (PCP'S) OFFICE...
HE WON'T EAT. HE'S LOST 25 POUNDS...
HE'S SO SHAKY HE BROKE THE VASE HE WAS PAINTING.
HMM...
PCP
I'D LIKE TO RUN SOME TESTS.
WHAT ARE THEY SAYING?

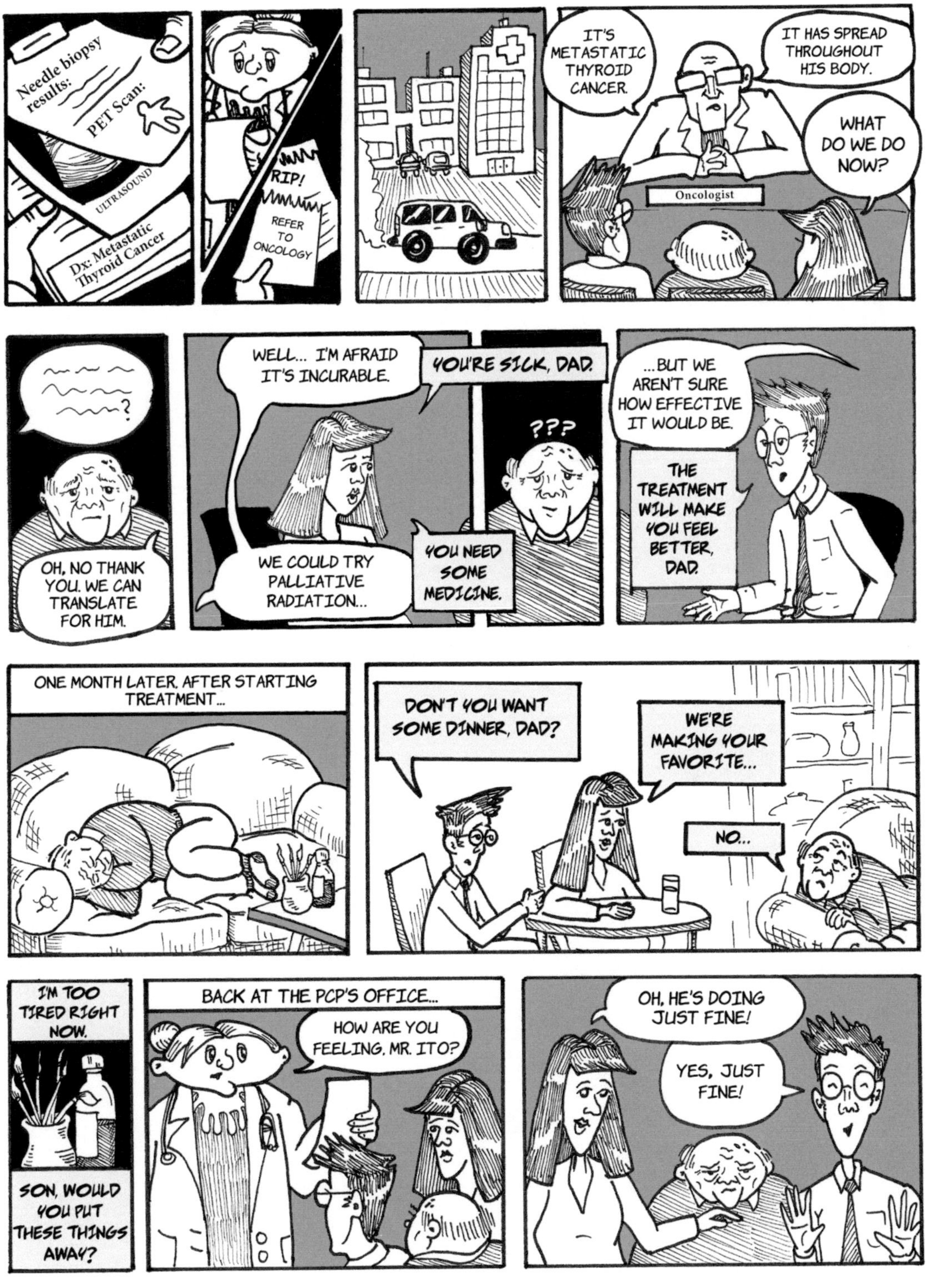
Needle biopsy results:
PET Scan:
ULTRASOUND
Dx: Metastatic Thyroid Cancer
RIP!
REFER TO ONCOLOGY
IT'S METASTATIC THYROID CANCER.
IT HAS SPREAD THROUGHOUT HIS BODY.
Oncologist
WHAT DO WE DO NOW?
?
OH, NO THANK YOU. WE CAN TRANSLATE FOR HIM.
WELL... I'M AFRAID IT'S INCURABLE.
YOU'RE SICK, DAD.
WE COULD TRY PALLIATIVE RADIATION...
YOU NEED SOME MEDICINE.
???
...BUT WE AREN'T SURE HOW EFFECTIVE IT WOULD BE.
THE TREATMENT WILL MAKE YOU FEEL BETTER, DAD.
ONE MONTH LATER, AFTER STARTING TREATMENT...
DON'T YOU WANT SOME DINNER, DAD?
WE'RE MAKING YOUR FAVORITE...
NO...
I'M TOO TIRED RIGHT NOW.
SON, WOULD YOU PUT THESE THINGS AWAY?
BACK AT THE PCP'S OFFICE...
HOW ARE YOU FEELING, MR. ITO?
OH, HE'S DOING JUST FINE!
YES, JUST FINE!

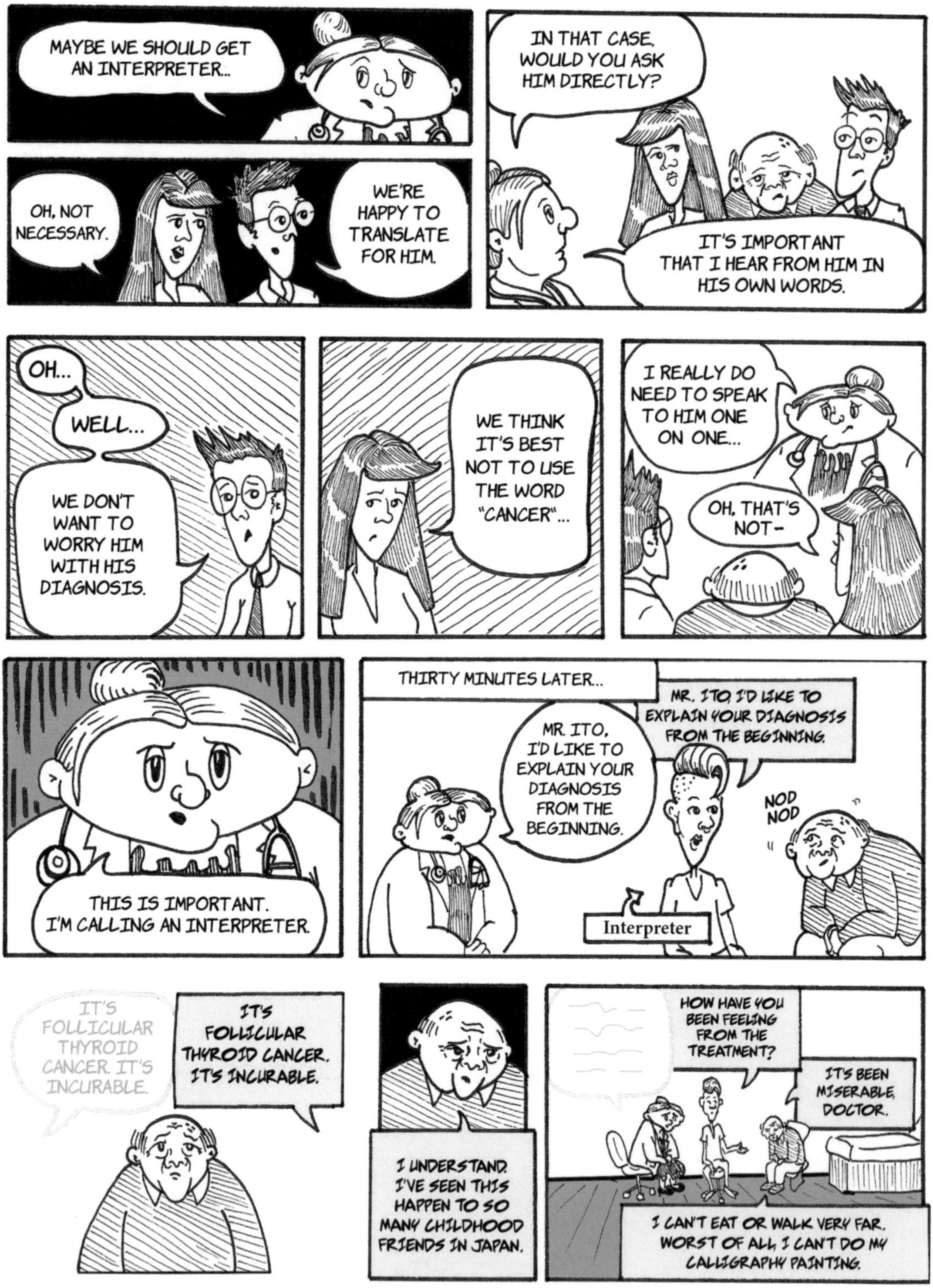
MAYBE WE SHOULD GET AN INTERPRETER...
OH, NOT NECESSARY.
WE'RE HAPPY TO TRANSLATE FOR HIM.
IN THAT CASE, WOULD YOU ASK HIM DIRECTLY?
IT'S IMPORTANT THAT I HEAR FROM HIM IN HIS OWN WORDS.
OH...
WELL...
WE DON'T WANT TO WORRY HIM WITH HIS DIAGNOSIS.
WE THINK IT'S BEST NOT TO USE THE WORD "CANCER"...
I REALLY DO NEED TO SPEAK TO HIM ONE ON ONE...
OH, THAT'S NOT-
THIS IS IMPORTANT. I'M CALLING AN INTERPRETER.
THIRTY MINUTES LATER...
MR. ITO, I'D LIKE TO EXPLAIN YOUR DIAGNOSIS FROM THE BEGINNING.
MR. ITO, I'D LIKE TO EXPLAIN YOUR DIAGNOSIS FROM THE BEGINNING.
NOD NOD
Interpreter
IT'S FOLLICULAR THYROID CANCER. IT'S INCURABLE.
IT'S FOLLICULAR THYROID CANCER. IT'S INCURABLE.
I UNDERSTAND. I'VE SEEN THIS HAPPEN TO SO MANY CHILDHOOD FRIENDS IN JAPAN.
HOW HAVE YOU BEEN FEELING FROM THE TREATMENT?
IT'S BEEN MISERABLE, DOCTOR.
I CAN'T EAT OR WALK VERY FAR. WORST OF ALL, I CAN'T DO MY CALLIGRAPHY PAINTING.

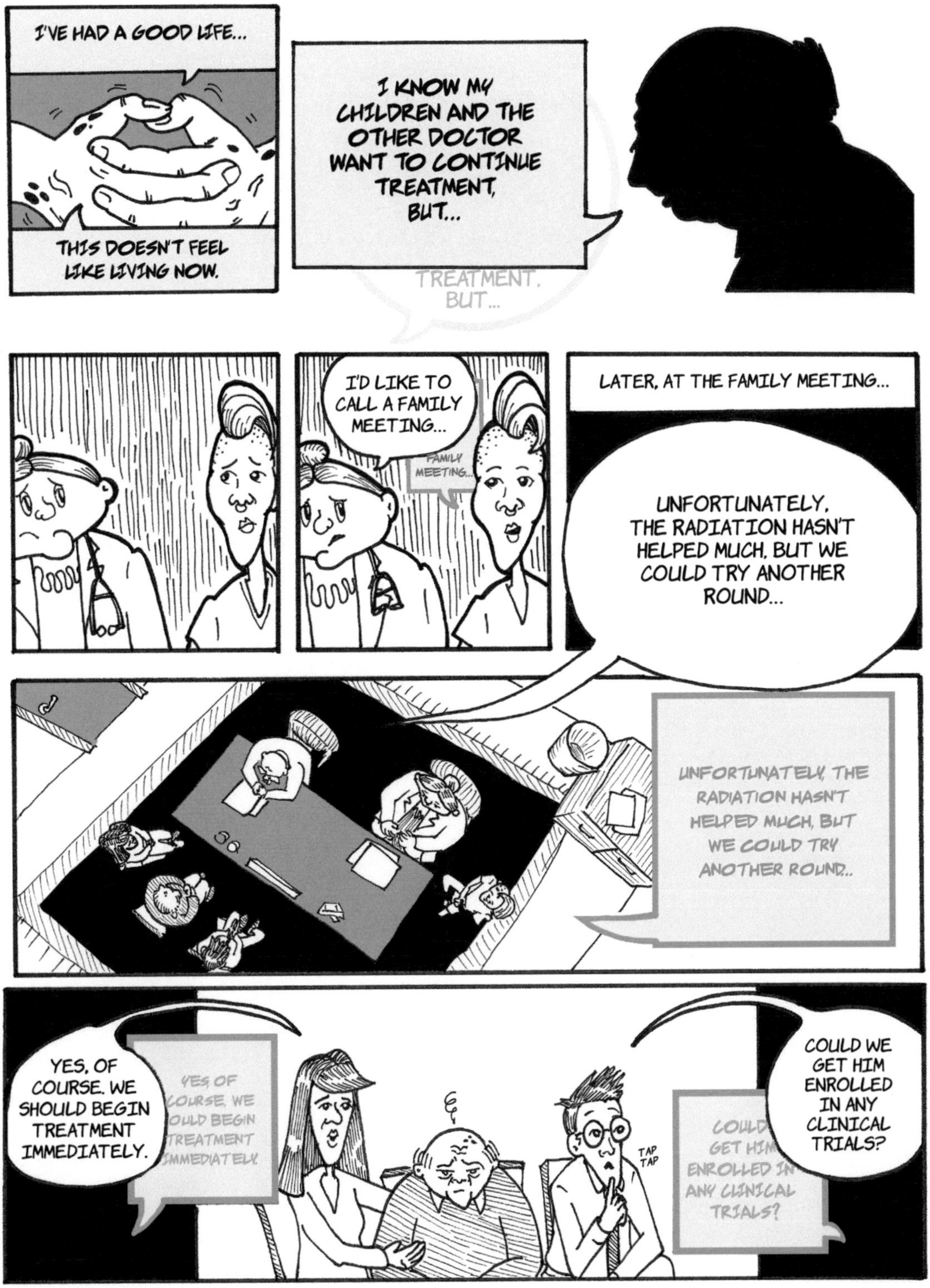
I'VE HAD A GOOD LIFE...
THIS DOESN'T FEEL LIKE LIVING NOW.
I KNOW MY CHILDREN AND THE OTHER DOCTOR WANT TO CONTINUE TREATMENT, BUT...
TREATMENT, BUT...
I'D LIKE TO CALL A FAMILY MEETING...
FAMILY MEETING...
LATER, AT THE FAMILY MEETING...
UNFORTUNATELY, THE RADIATION HASN'T HELPED MUCH, BUT WE COULD TRY ANOTHER ROUND...
UNFORTUNATELY, THE RADIATION HASN'T HELPED MUCH, BUT WE COULD TRY ANOTHER ROUND..
YES, OF COURSE. WE SHOULD BEGIN TREATMENT IMMEDIATELY.
TAP TAP
COULD WE GET HIM ENROLLED IN ANY CLINICAL TRIALS?

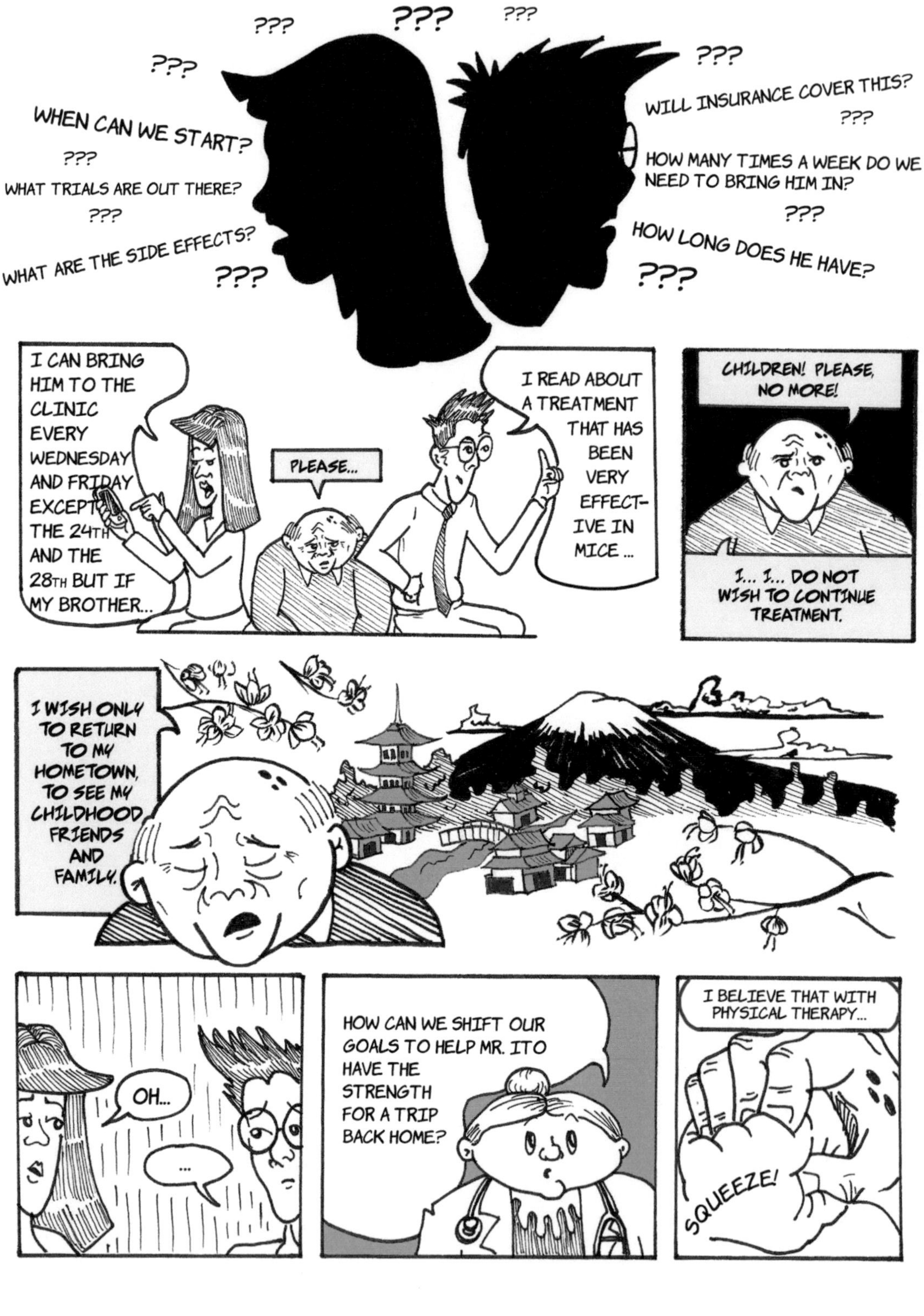
???
???
???
???
WHEN CAN WE START?
???
WHAT TRIALS ARE OUT THERE?
???
WHAT ARE THE SIDE EFFECTS?
???
???
WILL INSURANCE COVER THIS?
???
HOW MANY TIMES A WEEK DO WE NEED TO BRING HIM IN?
???
HOW LONG DOES HE HAVE?
???
I CAN BRING HIM TO THE CLINIC EVERY WEDNESDAY AND FRIDAY EXCEPT THE 24TH AND THE 28TH BUT IF MY BROTHER...
PLEASE...
I READ ABOUT A TREATMENT THAT HAS BEEN VERY EFFECT-IVE IN MICE ...
CHILDREN! PLEASE, NO MORE!
I... I... DO NOT WISH TO CONTINUE TREATMENT.
I WISH ONLY TO RETURN TO MY HOMETOWN, TO SEE MY CHILDHOOD FRIENDS AND FAMILY.
OH...
...
HOW CAN WE SHIFT OUR GOALS TO HELP MR. ITO HAVE THE STRENGTH FOR A TRIP BACK HOME?
I BELIEVE THAT WITH PHYSICAL THERAPY...
SQUEEZE!

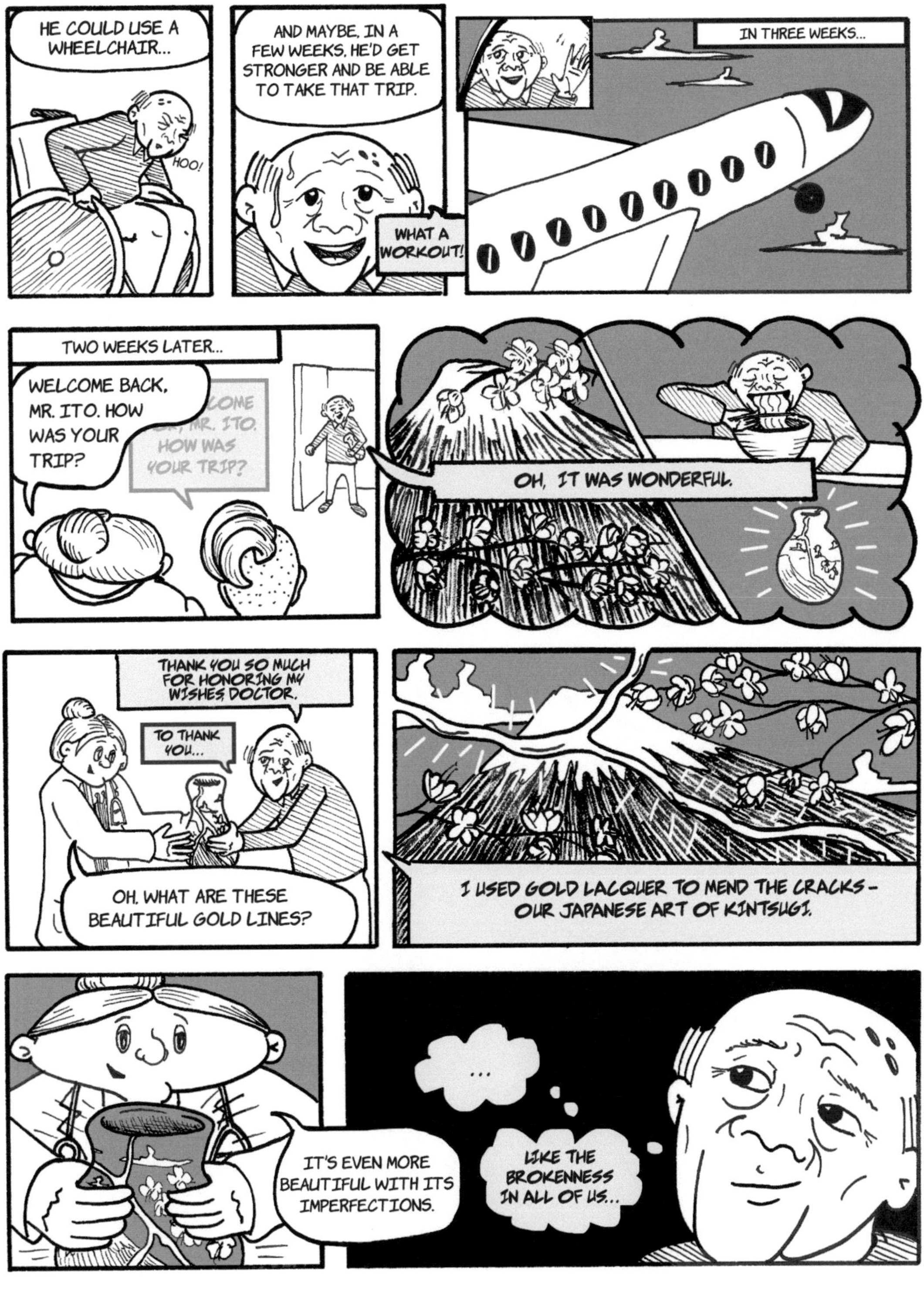
HE COULD USE A WHEELCHAIR...
HOO!
AND MAYBE, IN A FEW WEEKS, HE'D GET STRONGER AND BE ABLE TO TAKE THAT TRIP.
WHAT A WORKOUT!
IN THREE WEEKS...
TWO WEEKS LATER...
WELCOME BACK, MR. ITO. HOW WAS YOUR TRIP?
OH, IT WAS WONDERFUL.
THANK YOU SO MUCH FOR HONORING MY WISHES, DOCTOR.
TO THANK YOU...
OH, WHAT ARE THESE BEAUTIFUL GOLD LINES?
I USED GOLD LACQUER TO MEND THE CRACKS – OUR JAPANESE ART OF KINTSUGI.
IT'S EVEN MORE BEAUTIFUL WITH ITS IMPERFECTIONS.
...
LIKE THE BROKENNESS IN ALL OF US...

Discussion

Autonomy is a capacity to think and act freely, to make decisions for oneself and control one's own life. In order to exercise autonomy, a person must be free from controlling influences, including other people (well-meaning or not) and the withholding or selective sharing of information that a person would need in order to make independent medical decisions. To act autonomously, a person must understand a situation and be able to express how s/he wants to respond to it.

Healthcare providers' respect for patient autonomy is arguably the most highly honored of all ethical principles in twenty-first-century American medicine. Varying cultural contexts may, however, cause some patients to understand and practice autonomy in ways that differ from what healthcare providers might expect, and this discrepancy sometimes creates an ethical problem. *Broken Speech* illustrates some of the challenges that a family from a different culture—and their medical providers—might face in the U.S. medical system: conflicting approaches to learning and "breaking" bad news, differences in how individual autonomy is viewed, and difficulties navigating communication when a patient does not speak English.

Physicians in the United States consider it "best practice" to deliver important or difficult health news, such as a new diagnosis, to adult patients directly as an important way to respect their autonomy. The patient can ask that this information not be shared with anyone else, and such a request would be honored except in cases where health information must be reported (see also *Charting Courses*). In contrast to these norms, some cultures prefer that one's family be informed of an incurable cancer diagnosis *before* the patient is informed, as the person's health is relevant to the whole family. Because the Itos' cultural heritage deems it injurious to tell Mr. Ito that he has an incurable disease, his daughter and son withhold his true diagnosis while also supporting the oncologist's recommendation for radiation, believing that they are acting with beneficence by promoting Mr. Ito's physical and psychological well-being. From an ethical standpoint, however, they are disempowering their father because he does not know the facts he would want to know.

In the United States, it is typically assumed that individual patients will make their own medical decisions as long as they are of sound mind. As we see in *Broken Speech*, the Ito family's culture of origin again approaches things differently. The high value they place on interdependence and the whole family's or community's role in medical decision-making is not uncommon. It is shared by other groups within the United States—the Amish and Hasidic Jews, for instance—as well as other cultures around the world.

Complicating matters in this story is the fact that Mr. Ito does not understand or speak English well enough to comprehend medical information from his English-speaking doctors or to communicate his medical preferences so they are clearly understood. To respect a patient's autonomy fully, language barriers such as these should automatically trigger a request for an interpreter. However, this goal can be thwarted when an interpreter is not readily available (in a rural area, for instance) or compromised when well-meaning adult children, who are often already present in the room, offer to interpret. Even when certified medical interpreters are present, communication might not be fully accurate. This is particularly true with regard to nuances of breaking bad news about a complex diagnosis. After information has been translated, it is therefore important to ask the patient to explain in his or her own words what has been said to ensure that s/he has sufficiently grasped the situation.

When the primary care physician (PCP) in *Broken Speech* senses a significant breakdown in communication and insists on a medical interpreter, we learn that Mr. Ito does not in fact share his children's priorities, especially with regard to his continuing treatment. Finally able to assert his autonomy, Mr. Ito insists that quality of life is more important to him than quantity of life, and this declaration enables his healthcare team and his family to give him the one thing he desires most: to return home one last time.

It is important to note that a person's right to make autonomous medical decisions can extend to *not* wanting to know anything about his or her own diagnosis or medical progress. That is, a person can ask that information about his or her condition be shared only with a family member or friend, not directly with him or her. Members of the medical team are obligated to honor such a request even though it goes against their customary practice of full and direct disclosure to the patient. Such is the high value ascribed to patient autonomy.

A troubling barrier to autonomy is paternalism, any situation in which a physician or other healthcare professional overtly disregards or overrides a patient's wishes. Rarely is paternalism as simple as a physician's rejecting a patient's stated wish outright. Thanks to the news media, television shows, and social media, patients today are apt to know and assert their right to make autonomous decisions about their own healthcare in consultation with their doctors. Still, this ideal of doctor-patient partnership in clinical medicine is compromised when, for instance, a patient is in some way disadvantaged—as with nonresident patients who are not fluent in the language or who have limited access to healthcare, or elderly patients who were raised in a time when "the doctor knows best" and a person simply "follows doctor's orders" instead of asking questions or, certainly, expressing disagreement. Healthcare professionals in these situations, like Mr. Ito's PCP, must take great care to ensure that patients clearly understand what's at stake with a diagnosis and their choices moving forward (see also *The Swan*). Even though the Ito siblings love their father very much and want to give him the longest life possible, and even though the prescribed treatment might accomplish this goal, Mr. Ito's PCP insists that he demonstrate understanding about his illness and treatment options. She realizes that she cannot make assumptions, no matter how well-intended they are. This commitment costs the patient, the family, and the healthcare team a great deal of time and effort, yet it is all in service of empowering Mr. Ito to articulate and act on his values. Anything less on the part of the PCP would be paternalism, and the last part of Mr. Ito's life would have been, by his own estimation, filled with more suffering and less joy.

It is worth noting that a healthcare provider certainly may encourage—even try to persuade—a patient to choose a particular course of action that has the greatest likelihood of healing. To do so is to practice beneficence. Again, only if a physician were to manipulate a patient by withholding information, misrepresenting facts, and pressuring him would the physician be guilty of paternalistic behavior. In fact, and ironically, respecting a patient's autonomy can sometimes entail a physician's making decisions for the patient without much input from that patient—as in the example above of patients who do not want to know much about their medical condition, and when, for instance, they explicitly request that physicians make the best medically informed decisions on their behalf. Navigating these delicate boundaries is part of the art of medicine.

Questions for Further Reflection

1. What are some ways in which speech is broken in this comic?
2. Consider why Mr. Ito's children translate the oncologist's diagnosis and prognosis the way they do. What might have been their motivation to modify the information in this particular way? What about how they later report their father's progress to the primary care physician?
3. Contemplate the existential questions illustrated in this comic. What gives life meaning? What are some differences between curing and healing?
4. How does the art of kintsugi work as a metaphor within this story?
5. Explore in greater depth the following concepts related to autonomy: paternalism, decision-making capacity, patient competence.
6. Read Dax Cowart's story (Slotnik).

Related Readings

Annas, George J. "Informed Consent, Cancer, and Truth in Prognosis." *The Social Medicine Reader*, edited by Gail E. Henderson et al., Duke UP, 1997, pp. 341–46.

Barsky, Arthur J. "The Iatrogenic Potential of the Physician's Words." *Journal of the American Medical Association*, vol. 318, no. 24, 2017, pp. 2425–26.

Grouse, Lawrence D. "The Lie." *The Social Medicine Reader: Patients, Doctors, and Illness*, edited by Nancy M. P. King et al., Duke UP, 2005, pp. 205–7.

Orr, Robert. "Confessions of a Closet Paternalist." *The Western Journal of Medicine*, vol. 162, 1995, pp. 279–80.

Pellegrino, Edmund. "Is Truth-Telling to the Patient a Cultural Artifact?" *The Social Medicine Reader*, edited by Gail E. Henderson et al., Duke UP, 1997, pp. 330–32.

Pham, Kiemanh, et al. "Alterations During Medical Interpretation of ICU Family Conferences That Interfere with or Enhance Communication." *Chest*, vol. 134, no. 1, 2008, pp. 109–16.

Slotnik, Daniel E. "Dax Cowart, Who Suffered for Patients' Rights, Dies at 71." *New York Times*, 15 May 2019.

Wang, Lulu. *The Farewell*. Directed by Lulu Wang, Ray Productions et al., 2019.

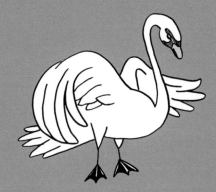

Chapter 2

Informed Consent

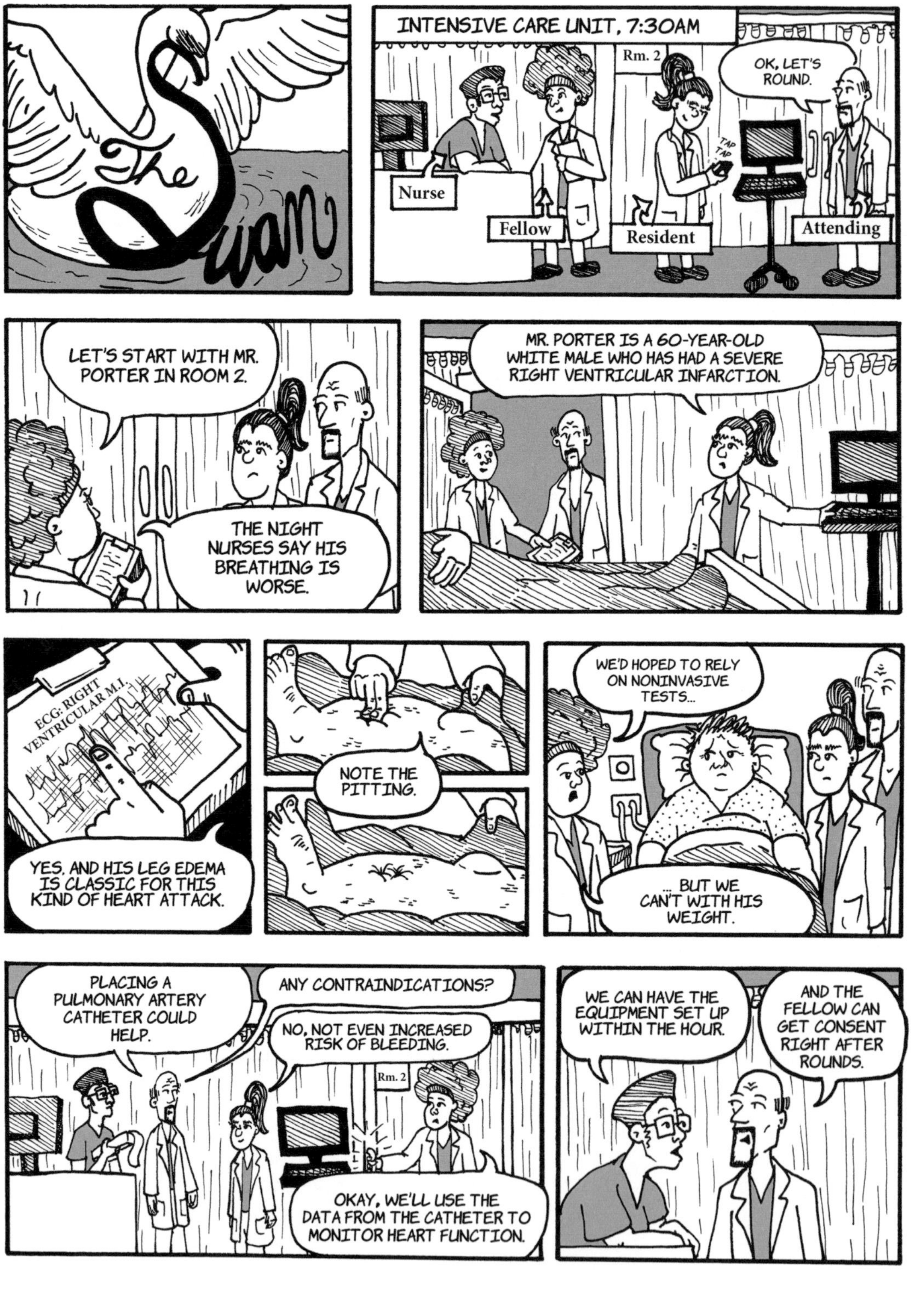
The Swan
INTENSIVE CARE UNIT, 7:30AM
Rm. 2
OK, LET'S ROUND.
TAP TAP
Nurse
Fellow
Resident
Attending
LET'S START WITH MR. PORTER IN ROOM 2.
THE NIGHT NURSES SAY HIS BREATHING IS WORSE.
MR. PORTER IS A 60-YEAR-OLD WHITE MALE WHO HAS HAD A SEVERE RIGHT VENTRICULAR INFARCTION.
ECG: RIGHT VENTRICULAR M.I.
YES. AND HIS LEG EDEMA IS CLASSIC FOR THIS KIND OF HEART ATTACK.
NOTE THE PITTING.
WE'D HOPED TO RELY ON NONINVASIVE TESTS...
... BUT WE CAN'T WITH HIS WEIGHT.
PLACING A PULMONARY ARTERY CATHETER COULD HELP.
ANY CONTRAINDICATIONS?
NO, NOT EVEN INCREASED RISK OF BLEEDING.
Rm. 2
OKAY, WE'LL USE THE DATA FROM THE CATHETER TO MONITOR HEART FUNCTION.
WE CAN HAVE THE EQUIPMENT SET UP WITHIN THE HOUR.
AND THE FELLOW CAN GET CONSENT RIGHT AFTER ROUNDS.

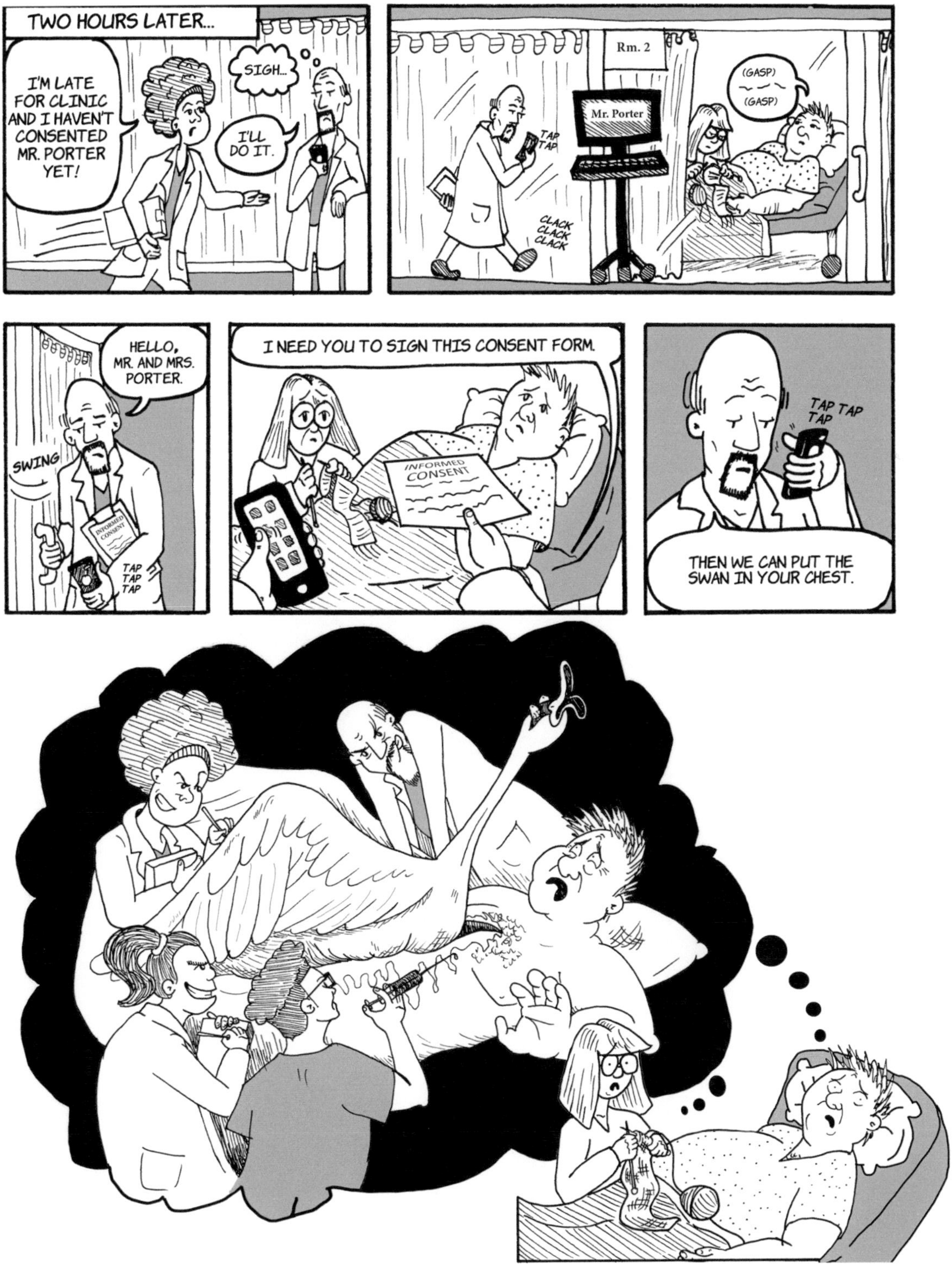
TWO HOURS LATER...
I'M LATE FOR CLINIC AND I HAVEN'T CONSENTED MR. PORTER YET!
SIGH...
I'LL DO IT.
Rm. 2
Mr. Porter
TAP TAP
(GASP) (GASP)
CLACK CLACK CLACK
HELLO, MR. AND MRS. PORTER.
SWING
INFORMED CONSENT
TAP TAP TAP
I NEED YOU TO SIGN THIS CONSENT FORM.
INFORMED CONSENT
TAP TAP TAP
THEN WE CAN PUT THE SWAN IN YOUR CHEST.

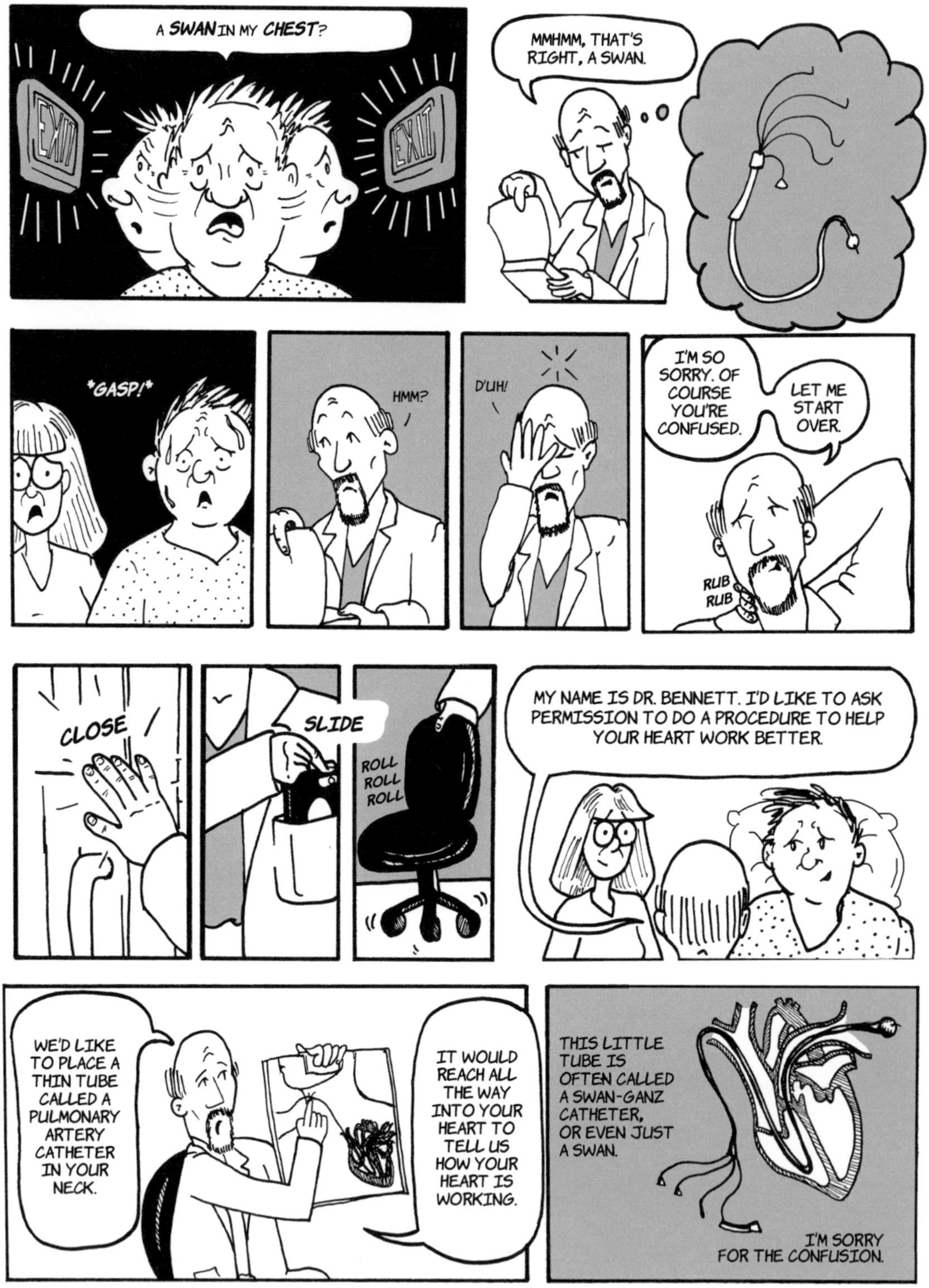
A SWAN IN MY CHEST?
EXIT
EXIT
MMHMM, THAT'S RIGHT, A SWAN.
GASP!
HMM?
D'UH!
I'M SO SORRY. OF COURSE YOU'RE CONFUSED.
LET ME START OVER.
RUB RUB
CLOSE
SLIDE
ROLL ROLL ROLL
MY NAME IS DR. BENNETT. I'D LIKE TO ASK PERMISSION TO DO A PROCEDURE TO HELP YOUR HEART WORK BETTER.
WE'D LIKE TO PLACE A THIN TUBE CALLED A PULMONARY ARTERY CATHETER IN YOUR NECK.
IT WOULD REACH ALL THE WAY INTO YOUR HEART TO TELL US HOW YOUR HEART IS WORKING.
THIS LITTLE TUBE IS OFTEN CALLED A SWAN-GANZ CATHETER, OR EVEN JUST A SWAN.
I'M SORRY FOR THE CONFUSION.

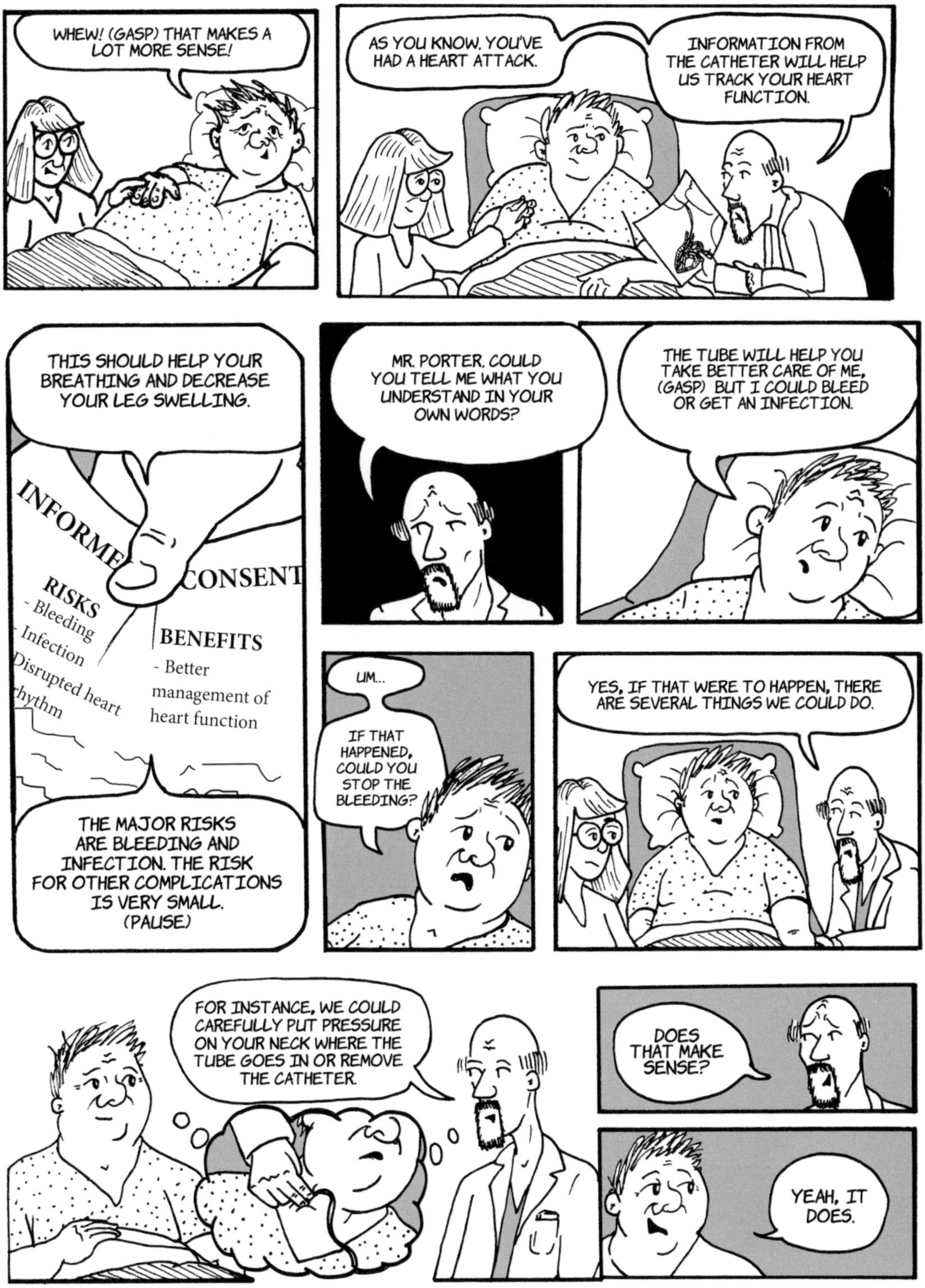
WHEW! (GASP) THAT MAKES A LOT MORE SENSE!
AS YOU KNOW, YOU'VE HAD A HEART ATTACK.
INFORMATION FROM THE CATHETER WILL HELP US TRACK YOUR HEART FUNCTION.
THIS SHOULD HELP YOUR BREATHING AND DECREASE YOUR LEG SWELLING.
INFORME CONSENT
RISKS
- Bleeding
- Infection
Disrupted heart rhythm
BENEFITS
- Better management of heart function
THE MAJOR RISKS ARE BLEEDING AND INFECTION. THE RISK FOR OTHER COMPLICATIONS IS VERY SMALL. (PAUSE)
MR. PORTER, COULD YOU TELL ME WHAT YOU UNDERSTAND IN YOUR OWN WORDS?
THE TUBE WILL HELP YOU TAKE BETTER CARE OF ME, (GASP) BUT I COULD BLEED OR GET AN INFECTION.
UM...
IF THAT HAPPENED, COULD YOU STOP THE BLEEDING?
YES, IF THAT WERE TO HAPPEN, THERE ARE SEVERAL THINGS WE COULD DO.
FOR INSTANCE, WE COULD CAREFULLY PUT PRESSURE ON YOUR NECK WHERE THE TUBE GOES IN OR REMOVE THE CATHETER.
DOES THAT MAKE SENSE?
YEAH, IT DOES.

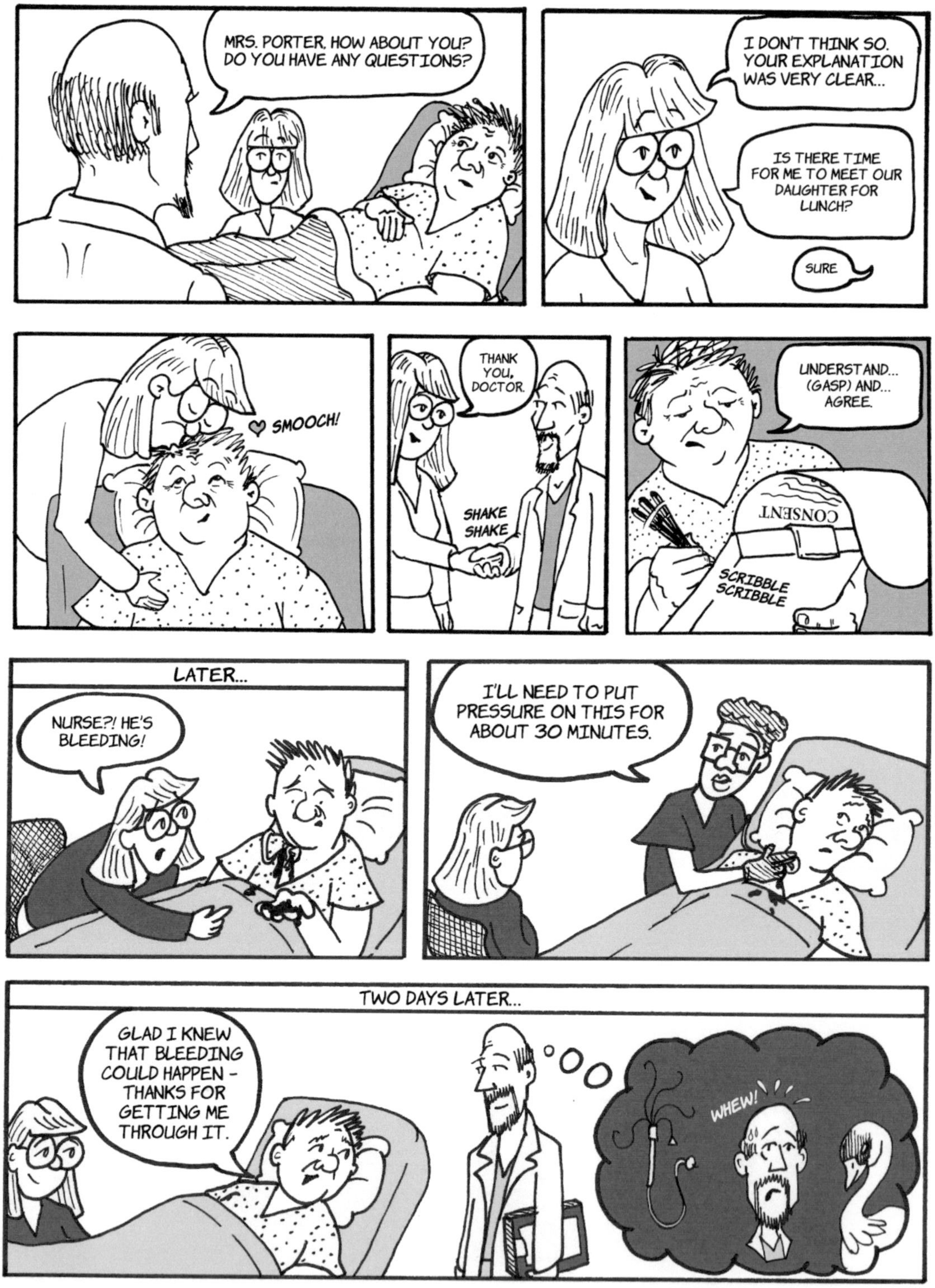
MRS. PORTER. HOW ABOUT YOU? DO YOU HAVE ANY QUESTIONS?
I DON'T THINK SO. YOUR EXPLANATION WAS VERY CLEAR...
IS THERE TIME FOR ME TO MEET OUR DAUGHTER FOR LUNCH?
SURE
SMOOCH!
THANK YOU, DOCTOR.
SHAKE SHAKE
UNDERSTAND... (GASP) AND... AGREE.
CONSENT
SCRIBBLE SCRIBBLE
LATER...
NURSE?! HE'S BLEEDING!
I'LL NEED TO PUT PRESSURE ON THIS FOR ABOUT 30 MINUTES.
TWO DAYS LATER...
GLAD I KNEW THAT BLEEDING COULD HAPPEN - THANKS FOR GETTING ME THROUGH IT.
WHEW!

When people hear the term "informed consent," they usually envision signing a form in order to receive medical care. But "getting consent" or "consenting the patient," as healthcare professionals often say, is more than just signing a form; it is a process that, when carried out appropriately, is an important educational moment that meets both legal and ethical standards for excellence in healthcare. *The Swan*, based on a true story, is a humorous example of the importance of fully informed consent, which may be defined as "a patient's willing acceptance of a medical intervention after a physician's adequate disclosure of the nature of the intervention, its risks, benefits, and alternatives."

A cornerstone of informed consent is respect for the patient's autonomy— ensuring the patient's right to determine what will be done with and to his or her own body. In order for the patient to make an autonomous decision, the diagnosis, and the justification for recommending a specific intervention (or "treatment") over other alternative interventions, must be explained in straightforward language. The healthcare professional must disclose the anticipated benefits and risks of the procedure as well as what might result *without* the intervention. Although this task might seem simple, it can often be fraught with pitfalls, some of which we see in *The Swan*.

How much to tell and how to tell it: Many medical procedures are complex. A person who has no medical training might not understand the details and implications of a proposed treatment. Therefore, the physician (or other designated provider) must determine which and how many details are necessary to share, and then must take great care to use language that the patient will accurately and fully comprehend. Translating intricate scientific, technological, and statistical information into clear language presents a challenge, especially given that the majority of Americans read between a sixth- and eighth-grade level and that healthcare professionals regularly use medical terminology among themselves for efficiency. Physicians must be sensitive to the fact that most patients won't understand medical terminology and that they may be confused or even frightened by such "jargon," as we see in Mr. and Mrs. Porter's situation.

A delicate balance: Determining how much information to discuss with the patient is part of the "art of medicine," the subjective aspects of clinical practice. A commonsense approach is to consider what is "reasonable" for both provider and patient: disclose as much as a reasonable practitioner would usually disclose according to customary practice, and as much as a reasonable person in the patient's position would consider relevant to his or her ability to make the right decision for him/herself. Bioethicist and family physician Howard Brody makes a good argument for what he calls the "transparency standard": providing as much information as is needed to render the physician's thought process clear and transparent to the patient (Brody 7). Especially because overall meaning can easily get lost in the midst of too many details, the transparency approach relieves a physician from the burden of trying to tease out every fact. To speak metaphorically here, the physician explains the tree with most of its branches; he does not discuss every leaf on the tree. In this way, providers can share what they are thinking and how they have reached a decision. Using visual images, as Dr. Bennett does in this vignette, can be particularly helpful.

Ask—tell—ask: Because the provider may not know what a patient understands even after a careful explanation, the provider should start the conversation by asking questions to determine what the patient knows already, what the patient hopes to accomplish, and what would be important for the patient to understand before undergoing a procedure. One helpful way to check for understanding is to ask the patient to explain the procedure in his or her own words. This provides space for further explanation and confirmation before the patient is asked to give consent for—or to refuse—treatment. Providers will often "ask—tell—ask": that is, ask (what does the patient know and what does the patient want to know)—tell (tell the patient what s/he needs to know)—and then ask again (ask the patient if s/he understands and what else s/he needs to know.

Questions for Further Reflection

1. What factors contribute to the Porters' initial misunderstanding? Consider factors related to the members of the medical team and to the Porters themselves.
2. Identify at least five concrete ways Dr. Bennett ultimately works to ensure that the Porters understand the proposed procedure.
3. How well does Dr. Bennett rectify his mistake once he realizes it? How does this situation impact the doctor-patient relationship immediately? After the procedure? How can you tell?
4. Think about how this story might impact your questions or comments the next time you or someone you love is "consented" for a medical intervention.

Related Readings

Basson, Marc D., Gerald Dworkin, and Eric J. Cassell. "Case Study: The 'Student Doctor' and a Wary Patient." *The Social Medicine Reader*, edited by Gail E. Henderson et al., Duke UP, 1997, pp. 323–26.

Brewster, Abenna. "A Student's View of a Medical Teaching Exercise." *The Social*

Medicine Reader, edited by Gail E. Henderson et al., Duke UP, 1997, pp. 236–37.

Brody, Howard. "Transparency: Informed Consent in Primary Care." *Hastings Center Report*, September/October 1989, pp. 5–9.

Gorovitz, Samuel. "Patient Autonomy." *Doctors' Dilemmas: Moral Conflict and Medical Care*, Macmillan, 1982, pp. 34–54.

Chapter 3 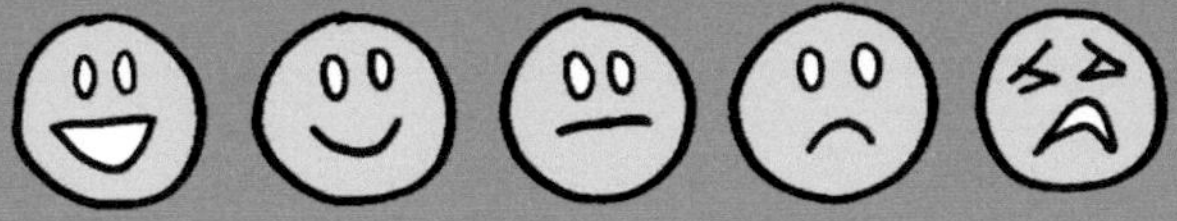

Unconscious Bias

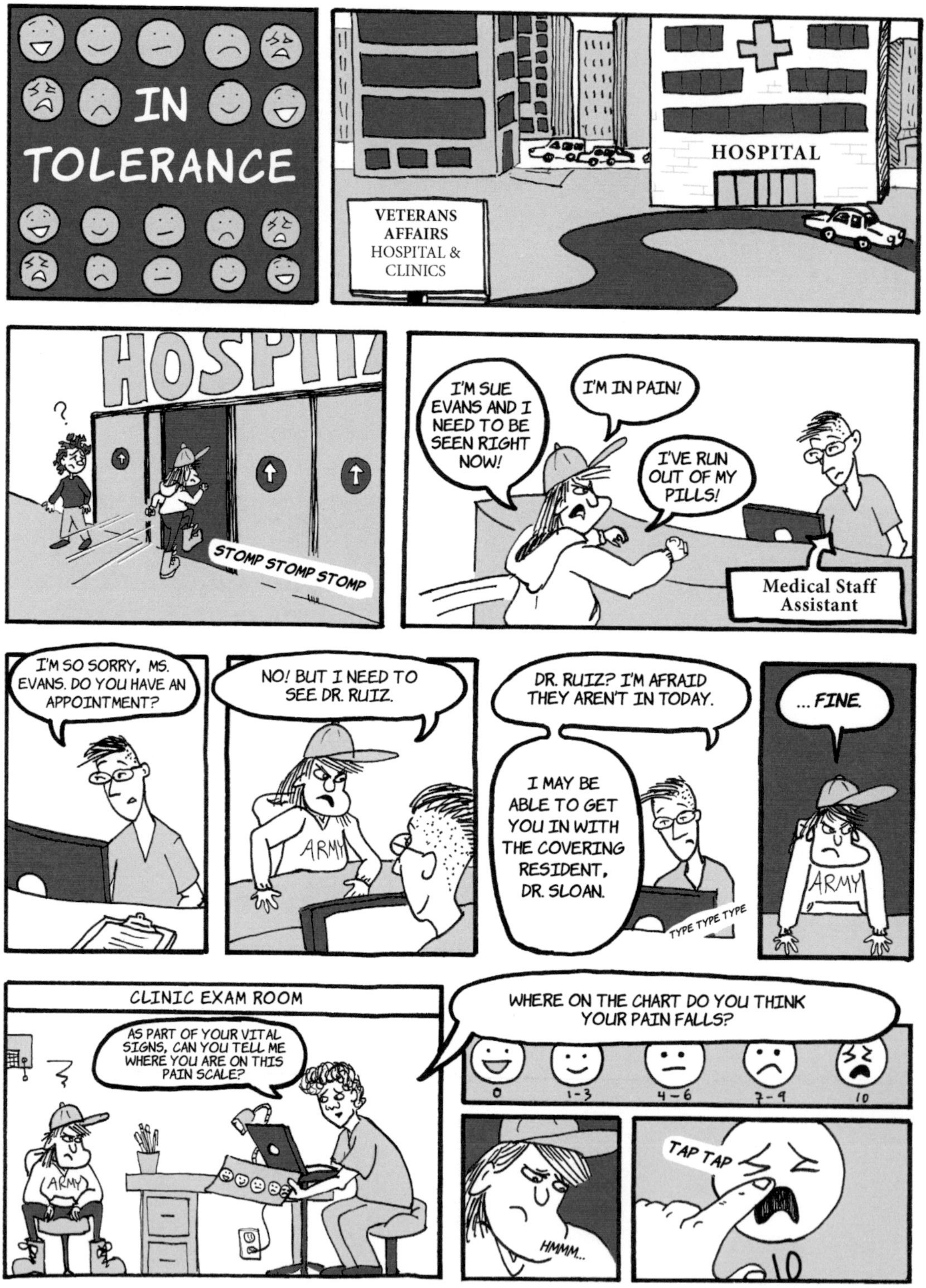
IN TOLERANCE
VETERANS AFFAIRS HOSPITAL & CLINICS
HOSPITAL
HOSPIT
?
STOMP STOMP STOMP
I'M SUE EVANS AND I NEED TO BE SEEN RIGHT NOW!
I'M IN PAIN!
I'VE RUN OUT OF MY PILLS!
Medical Staff Assistant
I'M SO SORRY, MS. EVANS. DO YOU HAVE AN APPOINTMENT?
NO! BUT I NEED TO SEE DR. RUIZ.
ARMY
DR. RUIZ? I'M AFRAID THEY AREN'T IN TODAY.
I MAY BE ABLE TO GET YOU IN WITH THE COVERING RESIDENT, DR. SLOAN.
TYPE TYPE TYPE
... FINE.
ARMY
CLINIC EXAM ROOM
AS PART OF YOUR VITAL SIGNS, CAN YOU TELL ME WHERE YOU ARE ON THIS PAIN SCALE?
ARMY
WHERE ON THE CHART DO YOU THINK YOUR PAIN FALLS?
0
1-3
4-6
7-9
10
HMMM...
TAP TAP
10

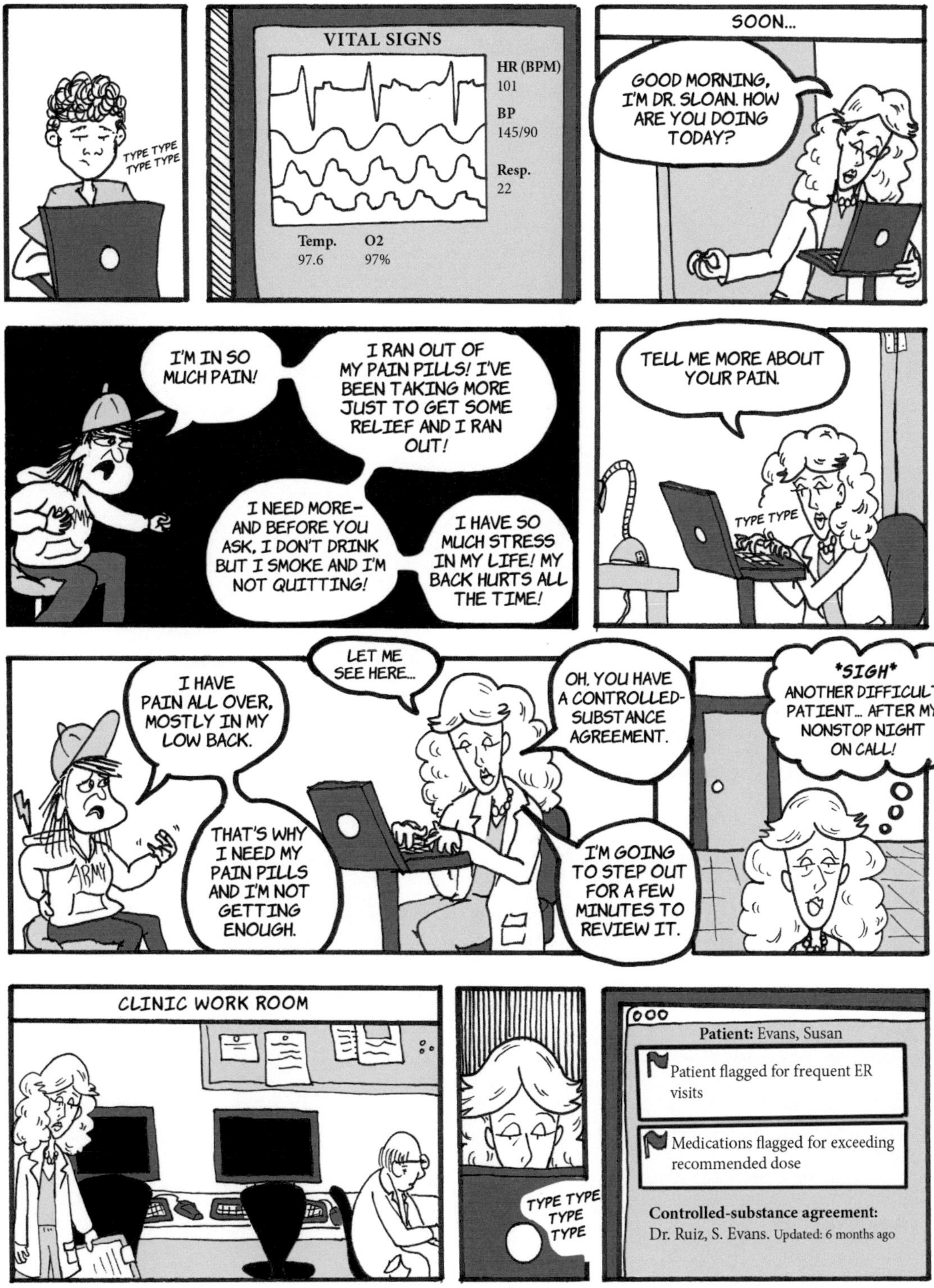
TYPE TYPE
TYPE TYPE
VITAL SIGNS
HR (BPM)
101
BP
145/90
Resp.
22
Temp.
97.6
O2
97%
SOON...
GOOD MORNING, I'M DR. SLOAN. HOW ARE YOU DOING TODAY?
I'M IN SO MUCH PAIN!
I RAN OUT OF MY PAIN PILLS! I'VE BEEN TAKING MORE JUST TO GET SOME RELIEF AND I RAN OUT!
I NEED MORE– AND BEFORE YOU ASK, I DON'T DRINK BUT I SMOKE AND I'M NOT QUITTING!
I HAVE SO MUCH STRESS IN MY LIFE! MY BACK HURTS ALL THE TIME!
TELL ME MORE ABOUT YOUR PAIN.
TYPE TYPE
I HAVE PAIN ALL OVER, MOSTLY IN MY LOW BACK.
THAT'S WHY I NEED MY PAIN PILLS AND I'M NOT GETTING ENOUGH.
LET ME SEE HERE...
OH, YOU HAVE A CONTROLLED-SUBSTANCE AGREEMENT.
I'M GOING TO STEP OUT FOR A FEW MINUTES TO REVIEW IT.
SIGH ANOTHER DIFFICULT PATIENT... AFTER MY NONSTOP NIGHT ON CALL!
CLINIC WORK ROOM
TYPE TYPE
TYPE
TYPE
Patient: Evans, Susan
Patient flagged for frequent ER visits
Medications flagged for exceeding recommended dose
Controlled-substance agreement:
Dr. Ruiz, S. Evans. Updated: 6 months ago

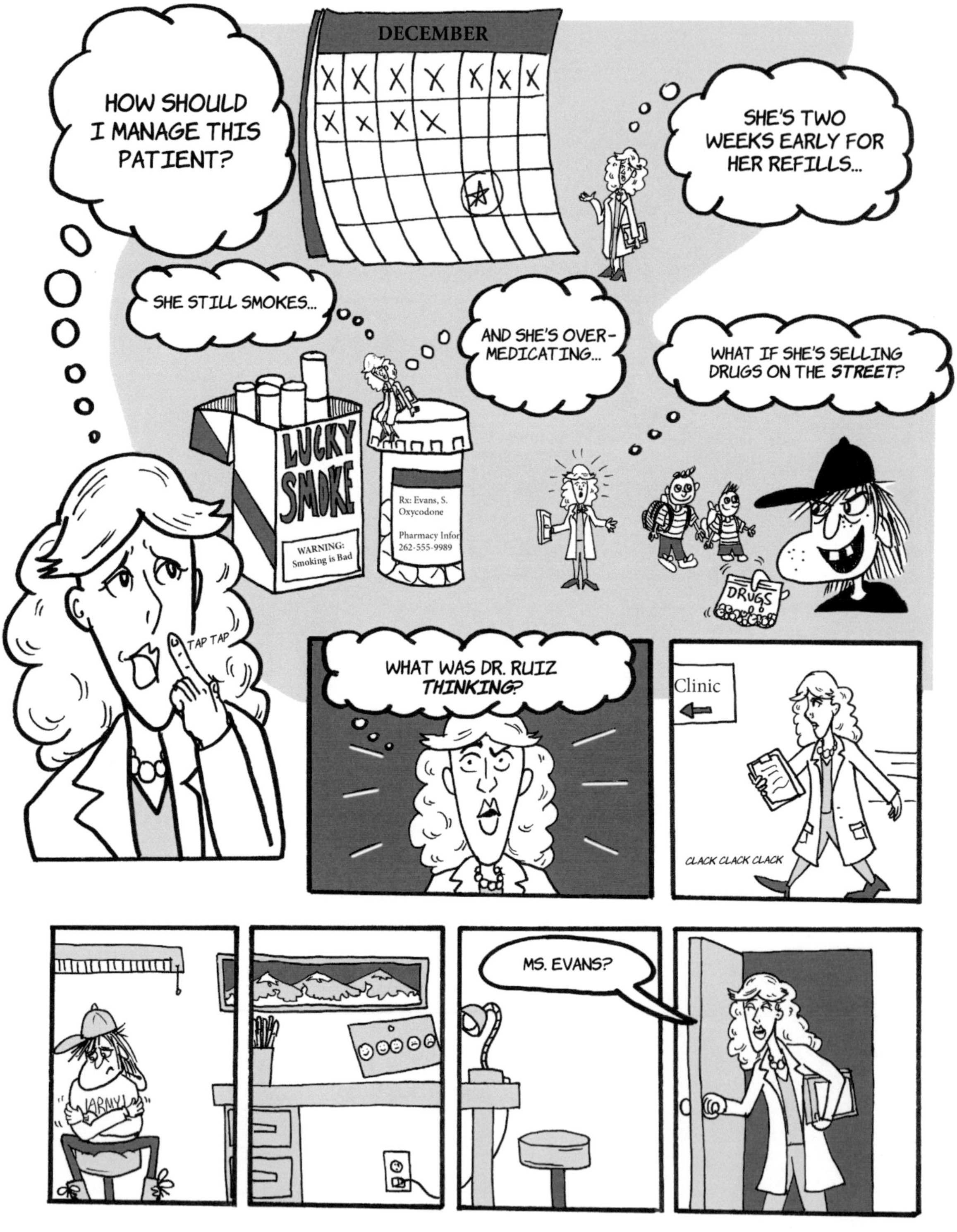
HOW SHOULD I MANAGE THIS PATIENT?
DECEMBER
SHE'S TWO WEEKS EARLY FOR HER REFILLS...
SHE STILL SMOKES...
AND SHE'S OVER-MEDICATING...
WHAT IF SHE'S SELLING DRUGS ON THE STREET?
LUCKY SMOKE
WARNING: Smoking is Bad
Rx: Evans, S.
Oxycodone
Pharmacy Infor
262-555-9989
DRUGS
TAP TAP
WHAT WAS DR. RUIZ THINKING?
Clinic
CLACK CLACK CLACK
ARMY
MS. EVANS?

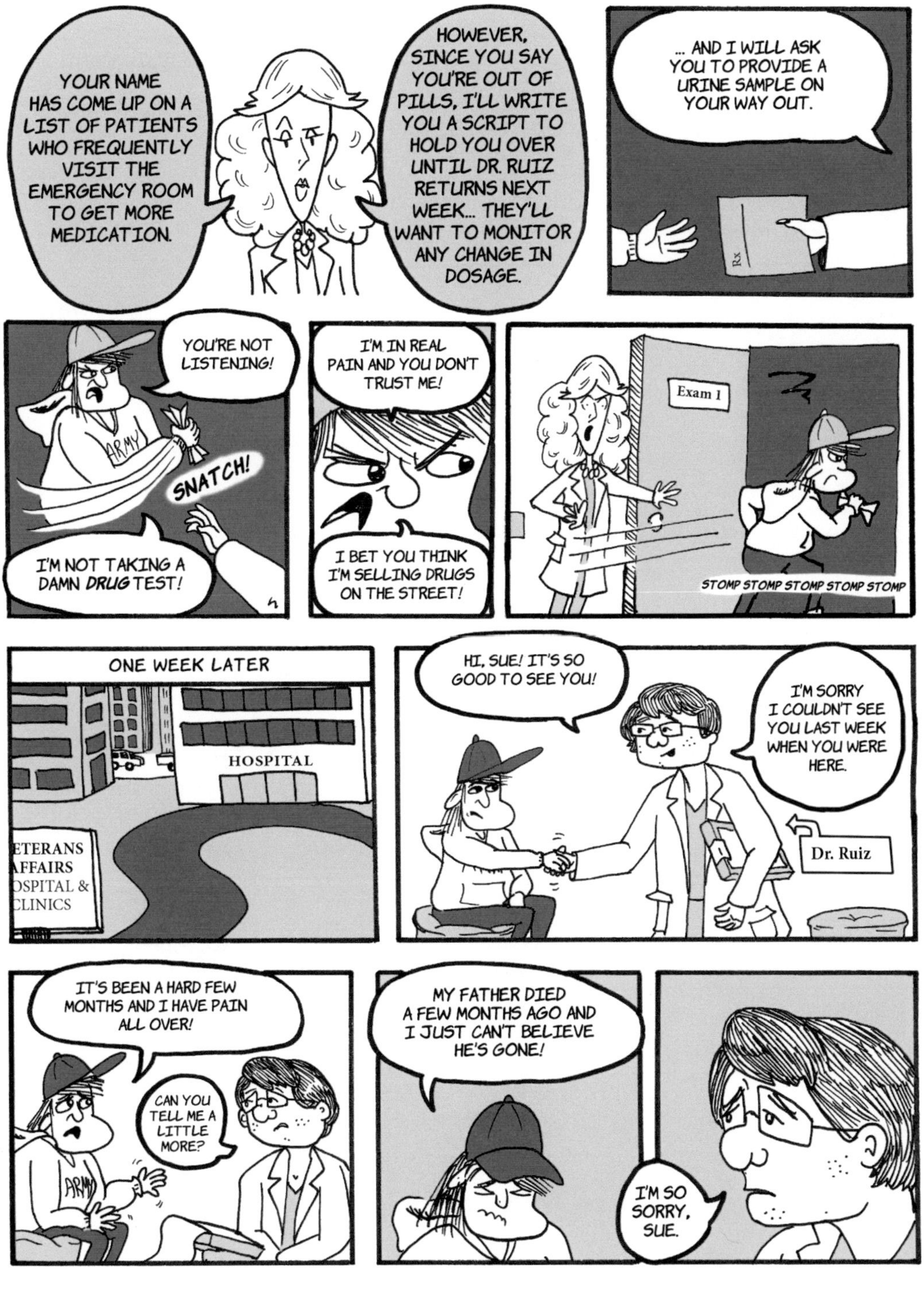
YOUR NAME HAS COME UP ON A LIST OF PATIENTS WHO FREQUENTLY VISIT THE EMERGENCY ROOM TO GET MORE MEDICATION.
HOWEVER, SINCE YOU SAY YOU'RE OUT OF PILLS, I'LL WRITE YOU A SCRIPT TO HOLD YOU OVER UNTIL DR. RUIZ RETURNS NEXT WEEK... THEY'LL WANT TO MONITOR ANY CHANGE IN DOSAGE.
... AND I WILL ASK YOU TO PROVIDE A URINE SAMPLE ON YOUR WAY OUT.
Rx
YOU'RE NOT LISTENING!
ARMY
SNATCH!
I'M NOT TAKING A DAMN DRUG TEST!
I'M IN REAL PAIN AND YOU DON'T TRUST ME!
I BET YOU THINK I'M SELLING DRUGS ON THE STREET!
Exam 1
STOMP STOMP STOMP STOMP STOMP
ONE WEEK LATER
HOSPITAL
ETERANS
AFFAIRS
OSPITAL &
CLINICS
HI, SUE! IT'S SO GOOD TO SEE YOU!
I'M SORRY I COULDN'T SEE YOU LAST WEEK WHEN YOU WERE HERE.
Dr. Ruiz
IT'S BEEN A HARD FEW MONTHS AND I HAVE PAIN ALL OVER!
CAN YOU TELL ME A LITTLE MORE?
ARMY
MY FATHER DIED A FEW MONTHS AGO AND I JUST CAN'T BELIEVE HE'S GONE!
I'M SO SORRY, SUE.

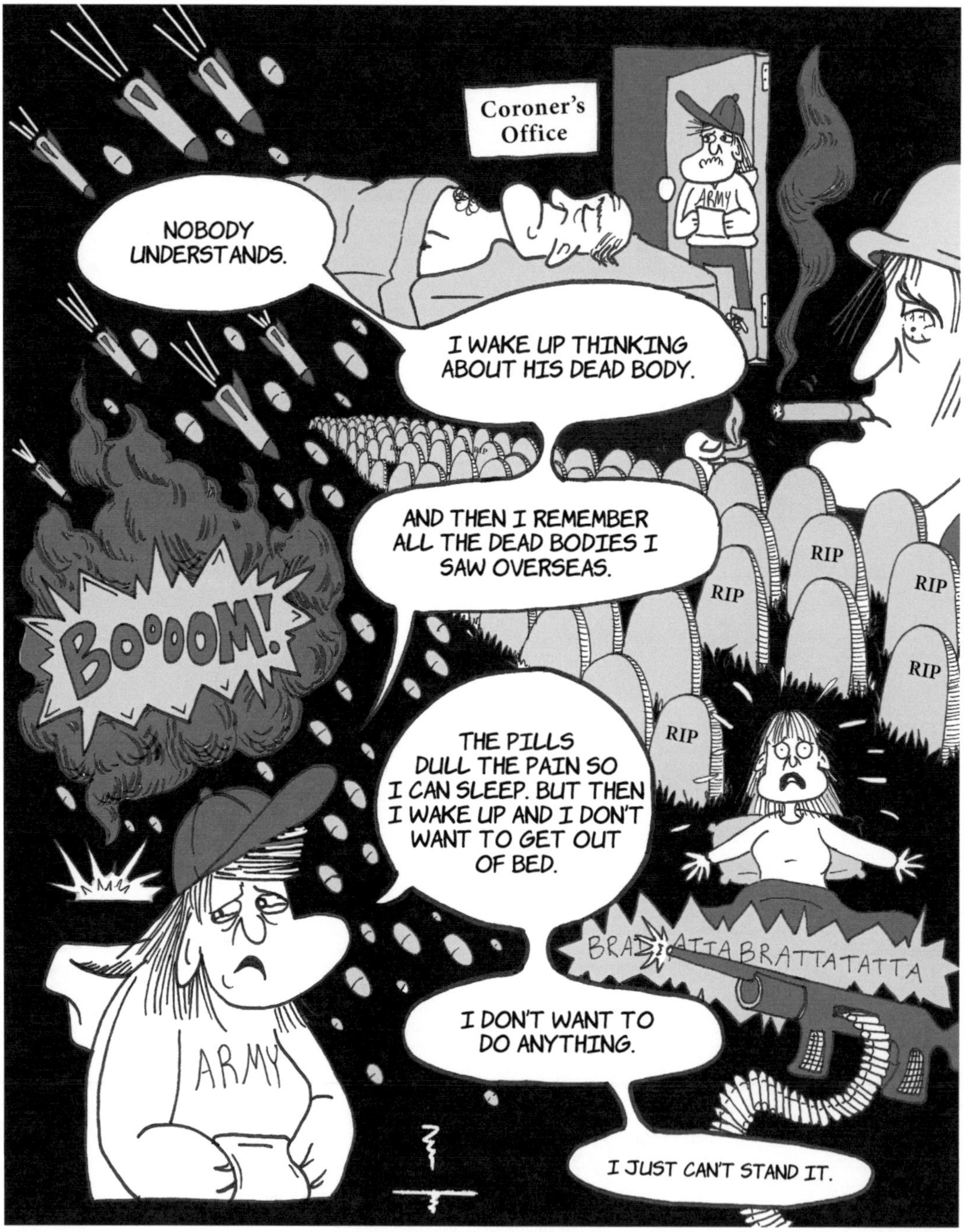
Coroner's Office
ARMY
NOBODY UNDERSTANDS.
I WAKE UP THINKING ABOUT HIS DEAD BODY.
AND THEN I REMEMBER ALL THE DEAD BODIES I SAW OVERSEAS.
BOoooOM!
RIP
THE PILLS DULL THE PAIN SO I CAN SLEEP. BUT THEN I WAKE UP AND I DON'T WANT TO GET OUT OF BED.
BRADATTABRATTATATTA
I DON'T WANT TO DO ANYTHING.
ARMY
I JUST CAN'T STAND IT.

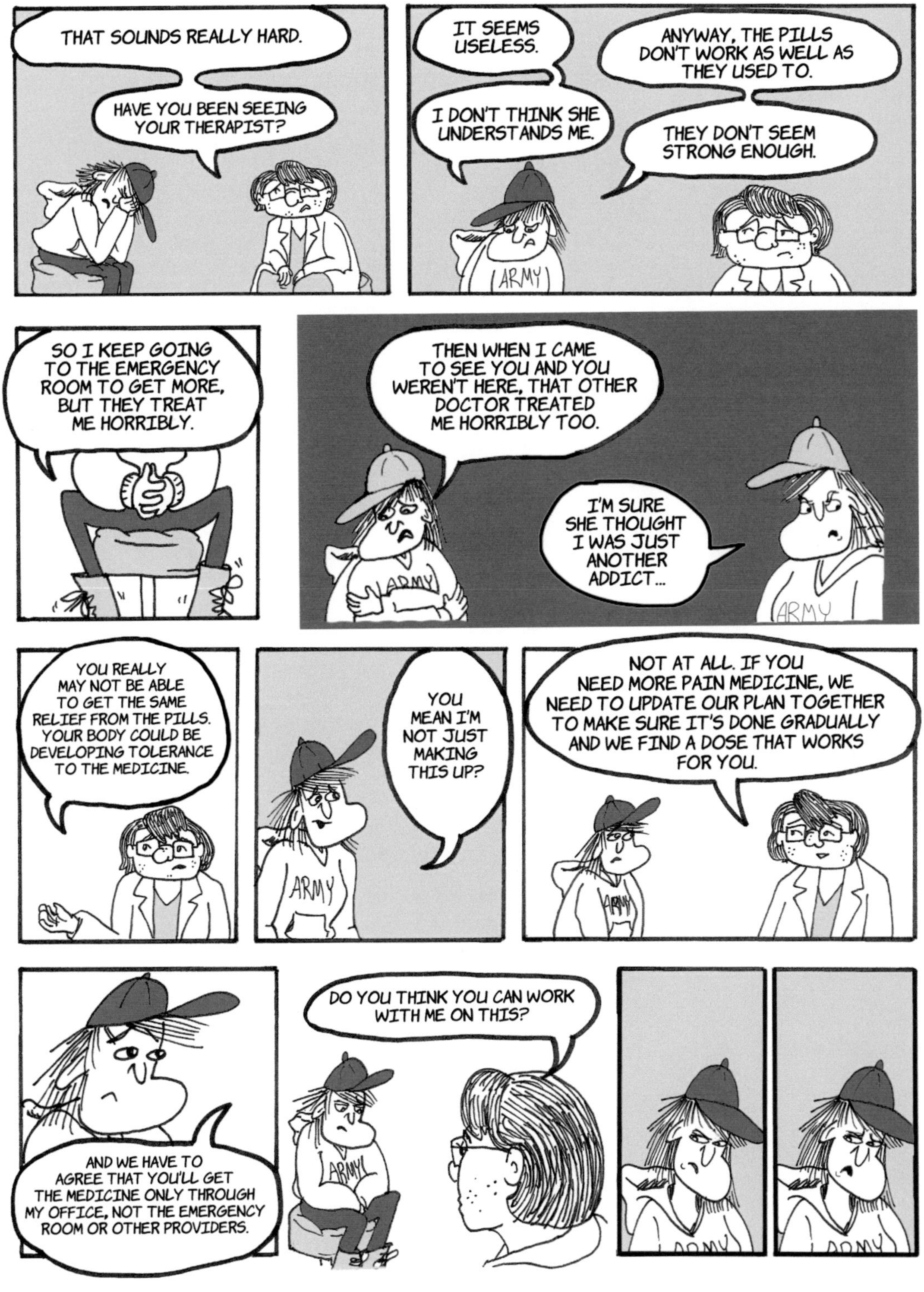
THAT SOUNDS REALLY HARD.
HAVE YOU BEEN SEEING YOUR THERAPIST?
IT SEEMS USELESS.
I DON'T THINK SHE UNDERSTANDS ME.
ANYWAY, THE PILLS DON'T WORK AS WELL AS THEY USED TO.
THEY DON'T SEEM STRONG ENOUGH.
ARMY
SO I KEEP GOING TO THE EMERGENCY ROOM TO GET MORE, BUT THEY TREAT ME HORRIBLY.
THEN WHEN I CAME TO SEE YOU AND YOU WEREN'T HERE, THAT OTHER DOCTOR TREATED ME HORRIBLY TOO.
I'M SURE SHE THOUGHT I WAS JUST ANOTHER ADDICT...
YOU REALLY MAY NOT BE ABLE TO GET THE SAME RELIEF FROM THE PILLS. YOUR BODY COULD BE DEVELOPING TOLERANCE TO THE MEDICINE.
YOU MEAN I'M NOT JUST MAKING THIS UP?
NOT AT ALL. IF YOU NEED MORE PAIN MEDICINE, WE NEED TO UPDATE OUR PLAN TOGETHER TO MAKE SURE IT'S DONE GRADUALLY AND WE FIND A DOSE THAT WORKS FOR YOU.
AND WE HAVE TO AGREE THAT YOU'LL GET THE MEDICINE ONLY THROUGH MY OFFICE, NOT THE EMERGENCY ROOM OR OTHER PROVIDERS.
DO YOU THINK YOU CAN WORK WITH ME ON THIS?

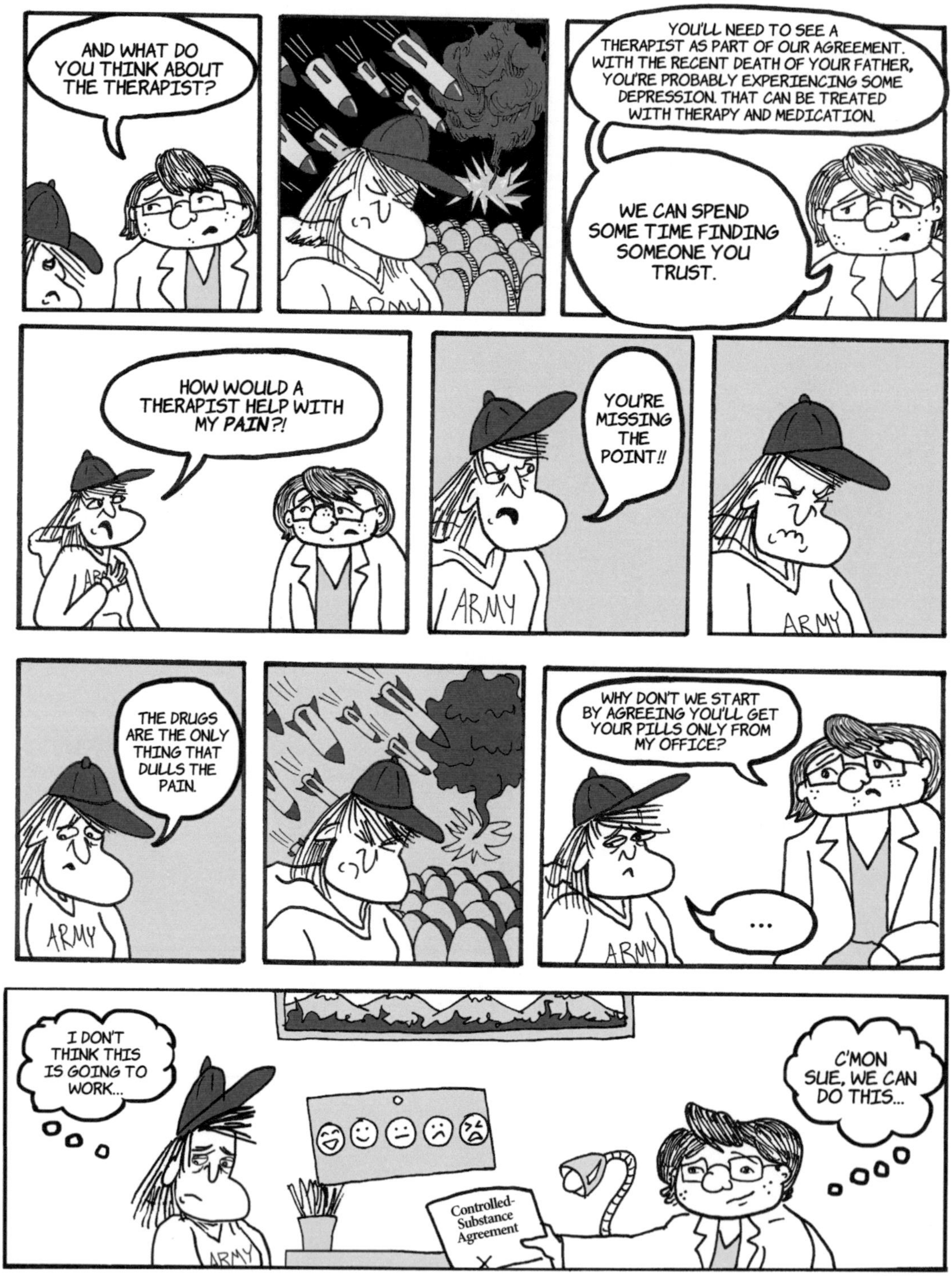
AND WHAT DO YOU THINK ABOUT THE THERAPIST?
YOU'LL NEED TO SEE A THERAPIST AS PART OF OUR AGREEMENT. WITH THE RECENT DEATH OF YOUR FATHER, YOU'RE PROBABLY EXPERIENCING SOME DEPRESSION. THAT CAN BE TREATED WITH THERAPY AND MEDICATION.
WE CAN SPEND SOME TIME FINDING SOMEONE YOU TRUST.
ARMY
HOW WOULD A THERAPIST HELP WITH MY **PAIN**?!
YOU'RE MISSING THE POINT!!
ARMY
ARMY
THE DRUGS ARE THE ONLY THING THAT DULLS THE PAIN.
ARMY
WHY DON'T WE START BY AGREEING YOU'LL GET YOUR PILLS ONLY FROM MY OFFICE?
...
ARMY
I DON'T THINK THIS IS GOING TO WORK...
C'MON SUE, WE CAN DO THIS...
Controlled-Substance Agreement
ARMY

Unconscious bias can occur when healthcare providers meet patients who are different from themselves in some way—in terms of, say, race, gender, ethnicity, or religion—or whose attitudes, behaviors, or lifestyles the physician may, consciously or not, consider questionable or harmful. Sue Evans's story tackles a hot-button issue for many healthcare providers: frustration with people who seem to want drugs to support an addiction rather than for a legitimate reason like acute, time-limited pain control. Such "drug-seeking behavior" raises red flags for providers not only for the irritation it causes but also because providers must be careful not to perpetuate phenomena like the opioid crisis of the 2020s.

Studies have shown that bias contributes to disparities in access to appropriate pain treatment between the "haves" and the "have-nots" (Passik and Kirsh). As a veteran who seems to be experiencing post-traumatic stress disorder (PTSD) and who may have difficulty holding a steady job, Sue presents as a "have-not." Her aggressiveness reinforces stereotypes about the behavior of patients who are seeking drugs due to an illness of addiction. When providers lose awareness of their automatic "gut responses" to patients with certain sociodemographic characteristics and/or vexing behavioral patterns, we call this prejudgment "unconscious bias."

In fact, unconscious bias can lead to substandard treatment (Marks and Sachar). When a patient's physical pain is not well controlled, other dimensions of suffering—including sleeplessness, fatigue, weight loss, anxiety, and depression—can emerge and contribute to a person's overall anguish. This cycle of undertreated pain has led Sue to a point of desperation, and Dr. Sloan's apparent dismissiveness only makes it worse. It seems to Sue as if she is being blamed for her own illness. She is caught in a vicious cycle. If she pushes too hard for her physician to treat her pain, her efforts may be construed as drug-seeking behavior. If she fails to convince her physician of the reality and severity of her pain, her physical distress will continue and her associated symptoms may worsen. Her physician's bias, therefore, forces Sue to choose between two inadequate and potentially humiliating choices.

Particularly in complex situations such as suspected drug-seeking behavior, it is essential for a physician to listen carefully to assess a patient for underlying "comorbidities," medical problems other than those for which the patient is presently being seen. For instance, although neither Dr. Sloan nor Dr. Ruiz mentions it, Sue's blood pressure (145/90) and heart rate (101) are a bit elevated. While these mild elevations could certainly be the result of Sue's general anxiety and the immediate tension caused by a clinic visit, Dr. Ruiz will likely keep these in mind, watching for trends in the wrong direction—trends that might suggest cardiac disease, for example. If appropriate, Dr. Ruiz can refer Sue to specialists, including pain management, physical therapy, or psychiatry, in order to manage symptoms more effectively and promote Sue's holistic well-being. And while Sue has signed a controlled-substance agreement in the past, Dr. Ruiz realizes they need to revisit it because Sue's situation has changed: she has likely developed tolerance to pain medication, and the death of her father has triggered emotional trauma.

A central feature of this comic is the importance of treating all patients with respect. Treating Sue with respect entails listening carefully and compassionately to her concerns, explaining why she might have developed tolerance to pain medication, and working with her to develop a controlled-substance agreement that provides relief while not promoting addiction. Such partnership between patient and doctor is vital to trust. In the end, the comic leaves us with the question "How can we act *in tolerance* instead of being *intolerant*?"

Questions for Further Reflection

1. What factors contribute to Dr. Sloan's initial impression that Sue Evans is seeking drugs to support an addiction? What about Sue might contribute to such an assumption? What about Dr. Sloan might contribute to such an assumption?

2. Why might certain populations—veterans, for example—carry unconscious biases toward medical providers and the healthcare system in general? Consider distrust of the medical profession as it exists in other marginalized populations whose past encounters have been ethically questionable or indeed patently unethical (e.g., Tuskegee).

3. Unconscious bias can go beyond the patient-doctor relationship. Consider situations where unconscious bias might be at play between physicians or between physicians and other hospital staff (e.g., Dr. Ruiz's nonbinary gender identity and the fact that they are Hispanic). How might this affect a patient's treatment?

4. What are some key components of a controlled-substance agreement? What might be some challenges to successful implementation of such an agreement?

5. Based on the conversation and the relationship between Sue and Dr. Ruiz, what is the likelihood that the new controlled-substance agreement will work?

6. Consider steps that healthcare providers—or anyone, for that matter— might take to guard against unconscious bias.

Baruch, Jay M. "Why Must Pain Patients Be Found Deserving of Treatment?" *Virtual Mentor*, vol. 10, no. 1, January 2008, pp. 5–12.

Cohen, Mitchell J., and William C. Jangro. "A Clinical Ethics Approach to Opioid Treatment of Chronic Noncancer Pain." *American Medical Association Journal of Ethics*, vol. 17, no. 6, 2015, pp. 521–29.

Marks, Richard M., and Edward J. Sachar. "Undertreatment of Medical Inpatients with Narcotic Analgesics." *Annals of Internal Medicine*, vol. 78, no. 2, 1973, pp. 173–81.

Passik, Steven D., and Kenneth L. Kirsh. "Double Standard for Access to Pain Management." *Virtual Mentor*, vol. 10, no. 1, January 2008, pp. 49–54.

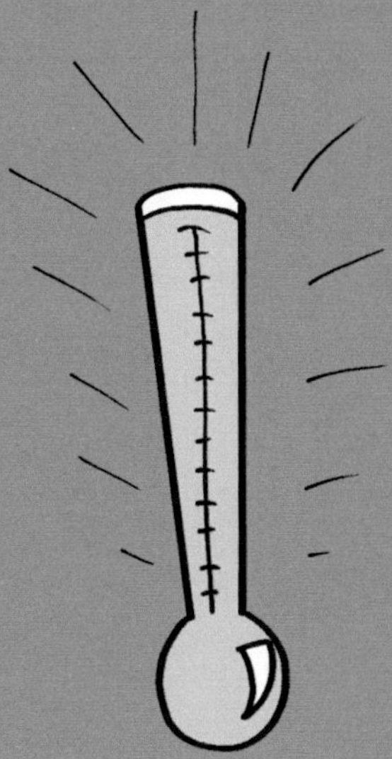

Chapter 4

Mandated Reporting of Suspected Abuse

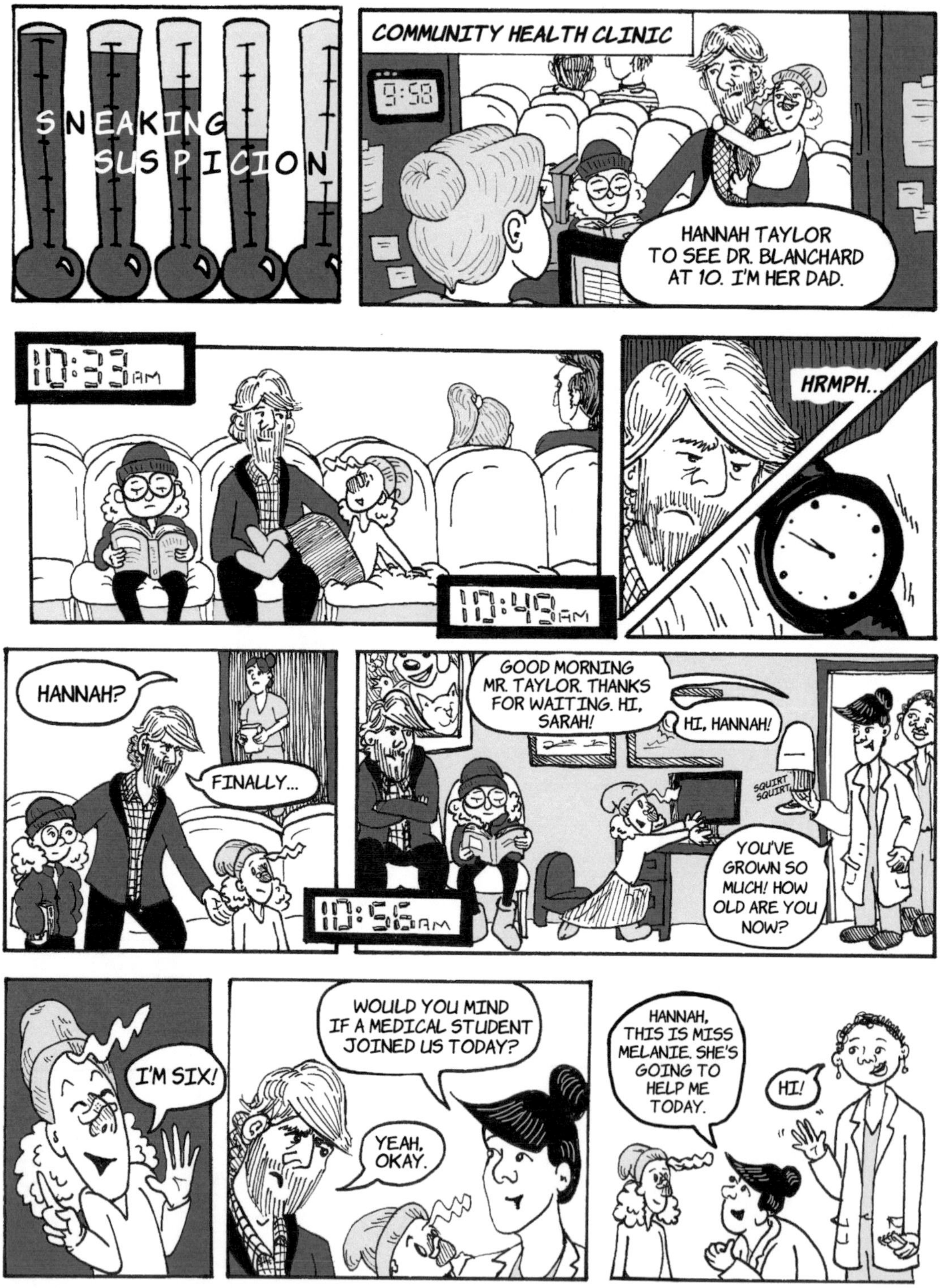
SNEAKING SUSPICION
COMMUNITY HEALTH CLINIC
9:58
HANNAH TAYLOR TO SEE DR. BLANCHARD AT 10. I'M HER DAD.
10:33 AM
10:49 AM
HRMPH...
HANNAH?
FINALLY...
10:55 AM
GOOD MORNING MR. TAYLOR. THANKS FOR WAITING. HI, SARAH!
HI, HANNAH!
SQUIRT SQUIRT
YOU'VE GROWN SO MUCH! HOW OLD ARE YOU NOW?
I'M SIX!
WOULD YOU MIND IF A MEDICAL STUDENT JOINED US TODAY?
YEAH, OKAY.
HANNAH, THIS IS MISS MELANIE. SHE'S GOING TO HELP ME TODAY.
HI!

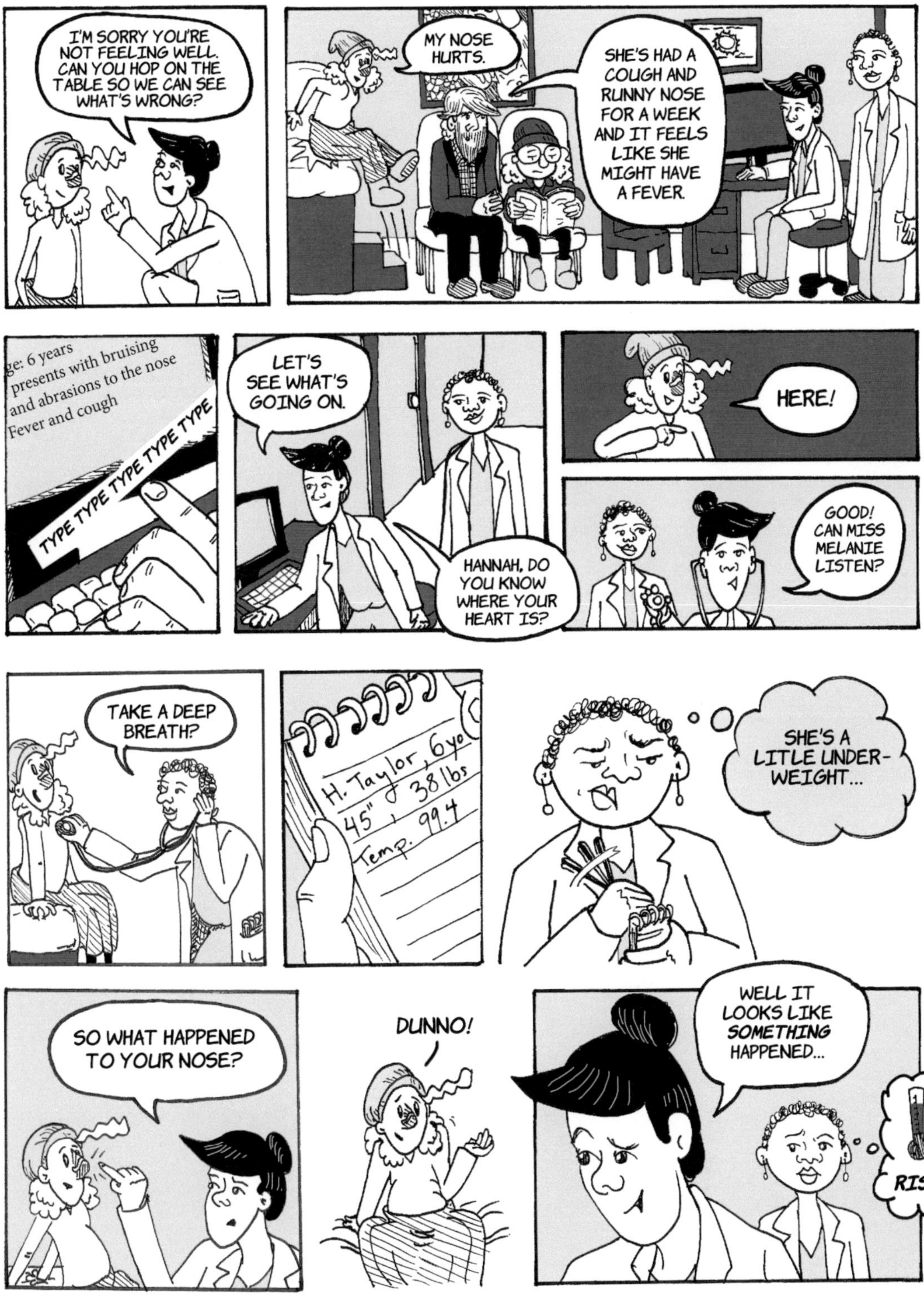
I'M SORRY YOU'RE NOT FEELING WELL. CAN YOU HOP ON THE TABLE SO WE CAN SEE WHAT'S WRONG?
MY NOSE HURTS.
SHE'S HAD A COUGH AND RUNNY NOSE FOR A WEEK AND IT FEELS LIKE SHE MIGHT HAVE A FEVER.
ge: 6 years
presents with bruising
and abrasions to the nose
Fever and cough
TYPE TYPE TYPE TYPE TYPE
LET'S SEE WHAT'S GOING ON.
HANNAH, DO YOU KNOW WHERE YOUR HEART IS?
HERE!
GOOD! CAN MISS MELANIE LISTEN?
TAKE A DEEP BREATH?
H. Taylor, 6yo
45" , 38 lbs
Temp. 99.4
SHE'S A LITTLE UNDER-WEIGHT...
SO WHAT HAPPENED TO YOUR NOSE?
DUNNO!
WELL IT LOOKS LIKE SOMETHING HAPPENED...
RISK?

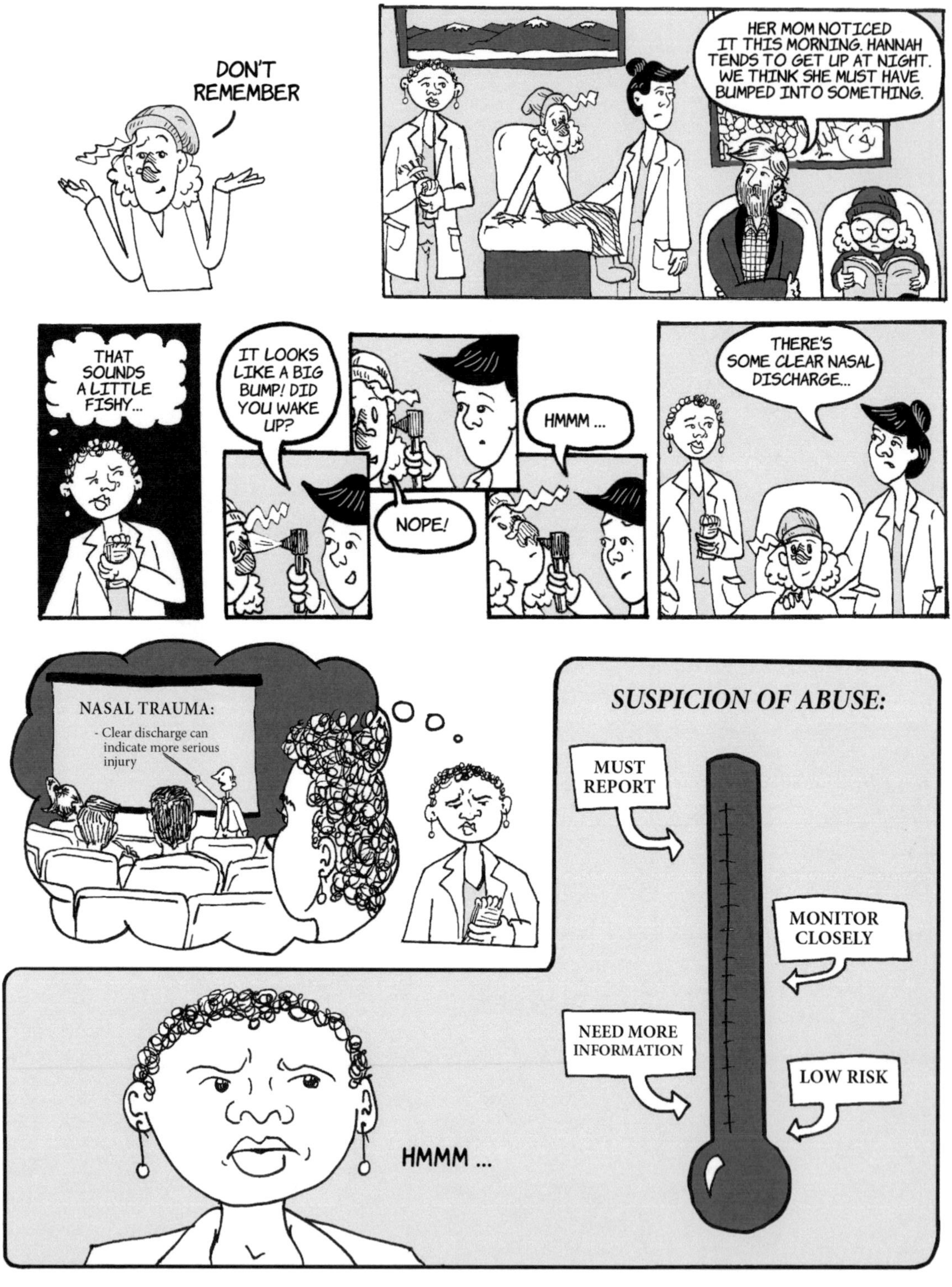
DON'T REMEMBER
HER MOM NOTICED IT THIS MORNING. HANNAH TENDS TO GET UP AT NIGHT. WE THINK SHE MUST HAVE BUMPED INTO SOMETHING.
THAT SOUNDS A LITTLE FISHY...
IT LOOKS LIKE A BIG BUMP! DID YOU WAKE UP?
NOPE!
HMMM ...
THERE'S SOME CLEAR NASAL DISCHARGE...
NASAL TRAUMA:
- Clear discharge can indicate more serious injury
SUSPICION OF ABUSE:
MUST REPORT
MONITOR CLOSELY
NEED MORE INFORMATION
LOW RISK
HMMM ...

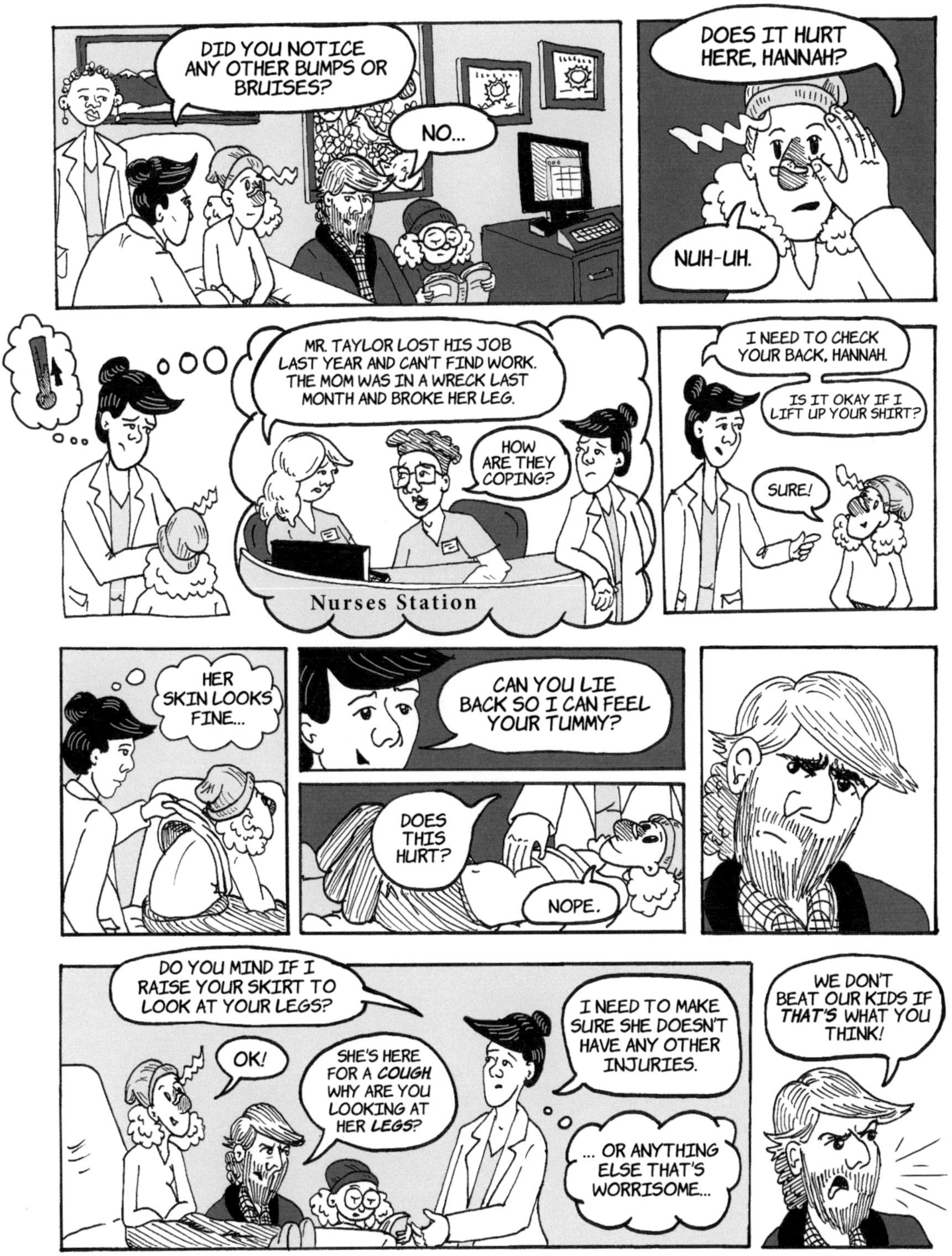
DID YOU NOTICE ANY OTHER BUMPS OR BRUISES?
NO...
DOES IT HURT HERE, HANNAH?
NUH-UH.
MR. TAYLOR LOST HIS JOB LAST YEAR AND CAN'T FIND WORK. THE MOM WAS IN A WRECK LAST MONTH AND BROKE HER LEG.
HOW ARE THEY COPING?
Nurses Station
I NEED TO CHECK YOUR BACK, HANNAH.
IS IT OKAY IF I LIFT UP YOUR SHIRT?
SURE!
HER SKIN LOOKS FINE...
CAN YOU LIE BACK SO I CAN FEEL YOUR TUMMY?
DOES THIS HURT?
NOPE.
DO YOU MIND IF I RAISE YOUR SKIRT TO LOOK AT YOUR LEGS?
OK!
SHE'S HERE FOR A COUGH. WHY ARE YOU LOOKING AT HER LEGS?
I NEED TO MAKE SURE SHE DOESN'T HAVE ANY OTHER INJURIES.
... OR ANYTHING ELSE THAT'S WORRISOME...
WE DON'T BEAT OUR KIDS IF THAT'S WHAT YOU THINK!

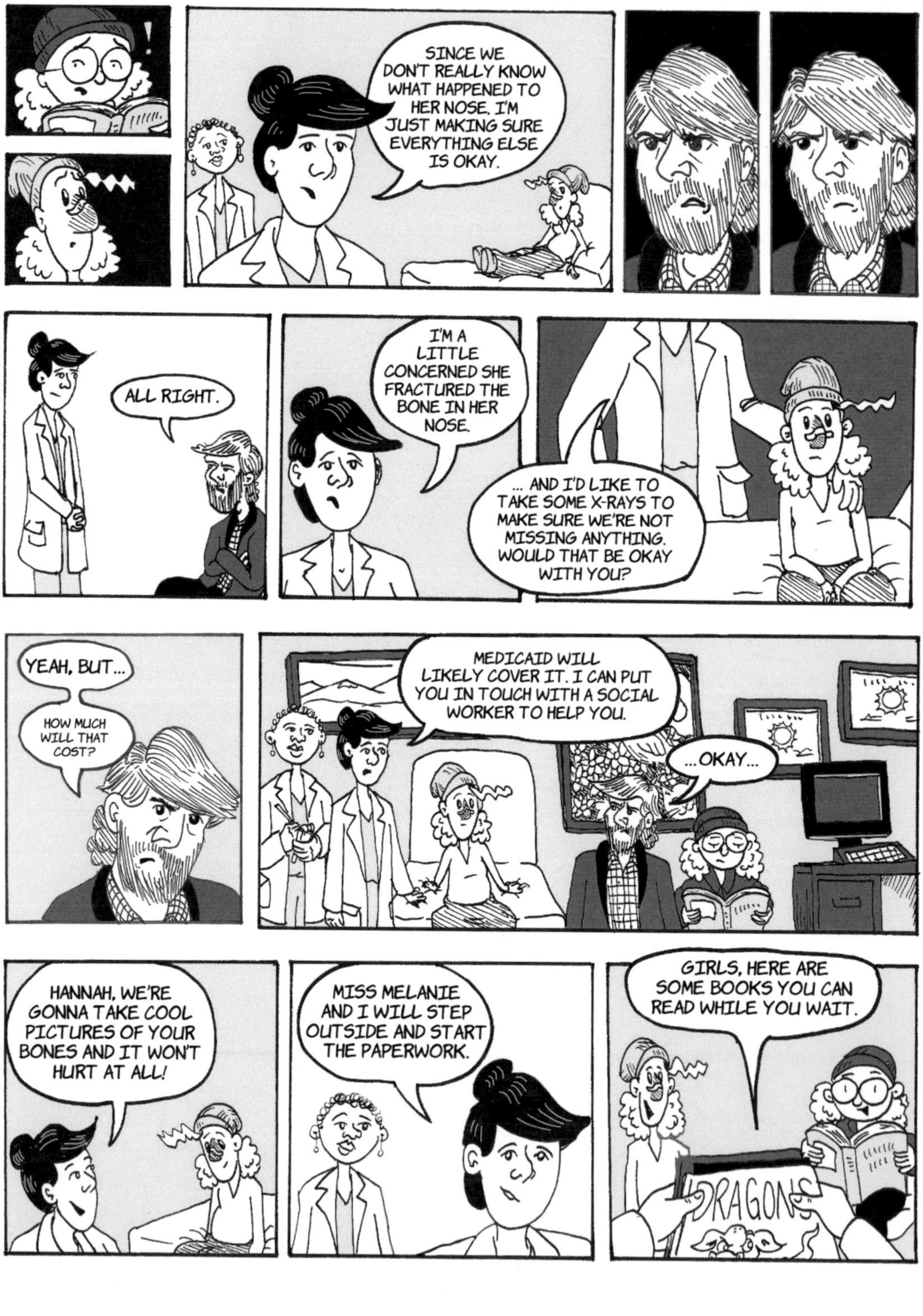
SINCE WE DON'T REALLY KNOW WHAT HAPPENED TO HER NOSE, I'M JUST MAKING SURE EVERYTHING ELSE IS OKAY.
ALL RIGHT.
I'M A LITTLE CONCERNED SHE FRACTURED THE BONE IN HER NOSE.
... AND I'D LIKE TO TAKE SOME X-RAYS TO MAKE SURE WE'RE NOT MISSING ANYTHING. WOULD THAT BE OKAY WITH YOU?
YEAH, BUT...
HOW MUCH WILL THAT COST?
MEDICAID WILL LIKELY COVER IT. I CAN PUT YOU IN TOUCH WITH A SOCIAL WORKER TO HELP YOU.
...OKAY...
HANNAH, WE'RE GONNA TAKE COOL PICTURES OF YOUR BONES AND IT WON'T HURT AT ALL!
MISS MELANIE AND I WILL STEP OUTSIDE AND START THE PAPERWORK.
GIRLS, HERE ARE SOME BOOKS YOU CAN READ WHILE YOU WAIT.
DRAGONS

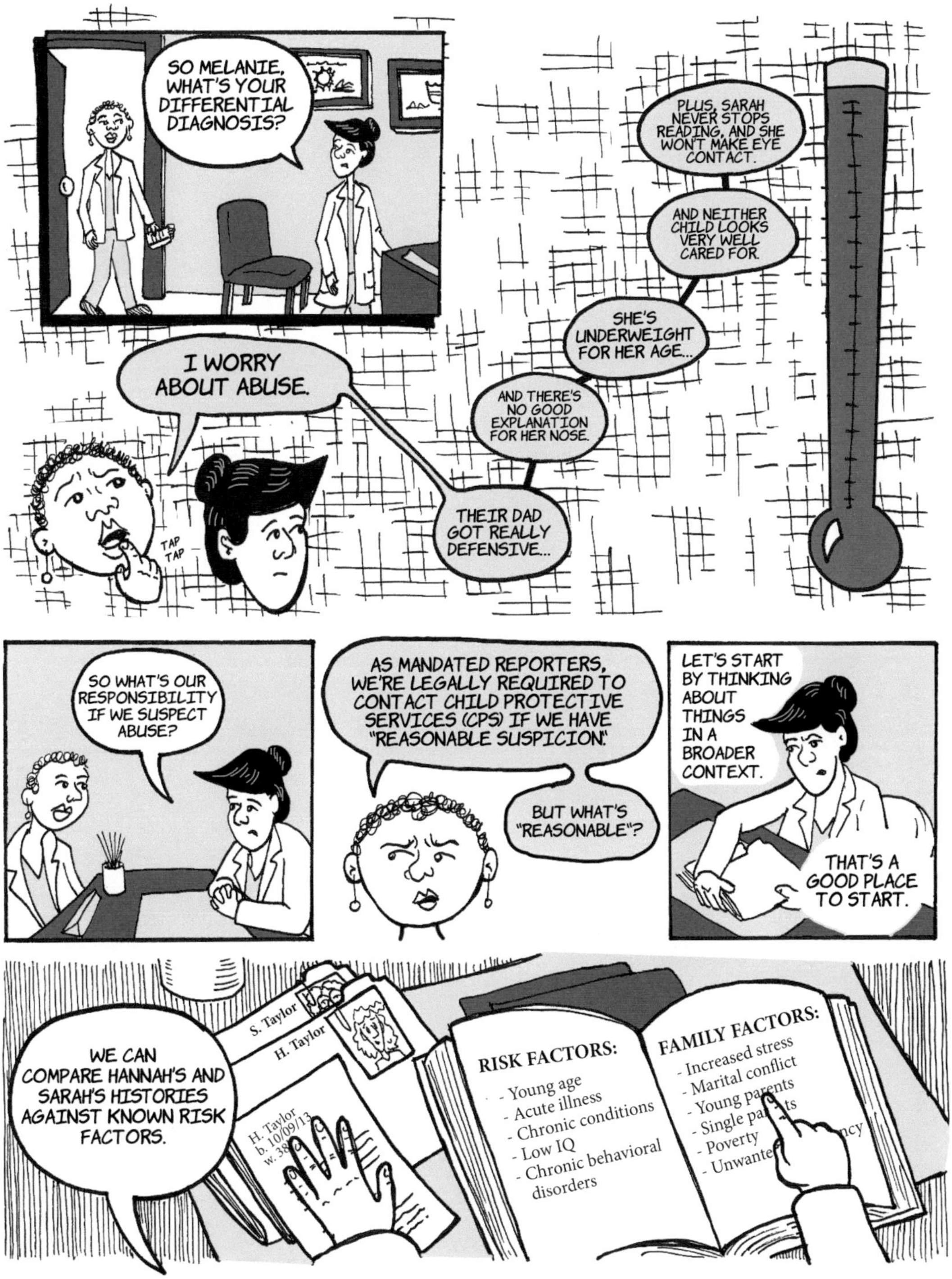
SO MELANIE, WHAT'S YOUR DIFFERENTIAL DIAGNOSIS?
I WORRY ABOUT ABUSE.
TAP TAP
THEIR DAD GOT REALLY DEFENSIVE...
AND THERE'S NO GOOD EXPLANATION FOR HER NOSE.
SHE'S UNDERWEIGHT FOR HER AGE...
AND NEITHER CHILD LOOKS VERY WELL CARED FOR.
PLUS, SARAH NEVER STOPS READING, AND SHE WON'T MAKE EYE CONTACT.
SO WHAT'S OUR RESPONSIBILITY IF WE SUSPECT ABUSE?
AS MANDATED REPORTERS, WE'RE LEGALLY REQUIRED TO CONTACT CHILD PROTECTIVE SERVICES (CPS) IF WE HAVE "REASONABLE SUSPICION."
BUT WHAT'S "REASONABLE"?
LET'S START BY THINKING ABOUT THINGS IN A BROADER CONTEXT.
THAT'S A GOOD PLACE TO START.
WE CAN COMPARE HANNAH'S AND SARAH'S HISTORIES AGAINST KNOWN RISK FACTORS.
S. Taylor
H. Taylor
H. Taylor
b. 10/09/13
RISK FACTORS:
- Young age
- Acute illness
- Chronic conditions
- Low IQ
- Chronic behavioral disorders
FAMILY FACTORS:
- Increased stress
- Marital conflict
- Young parents
- Single pa ts
- Poverty
- Unwante

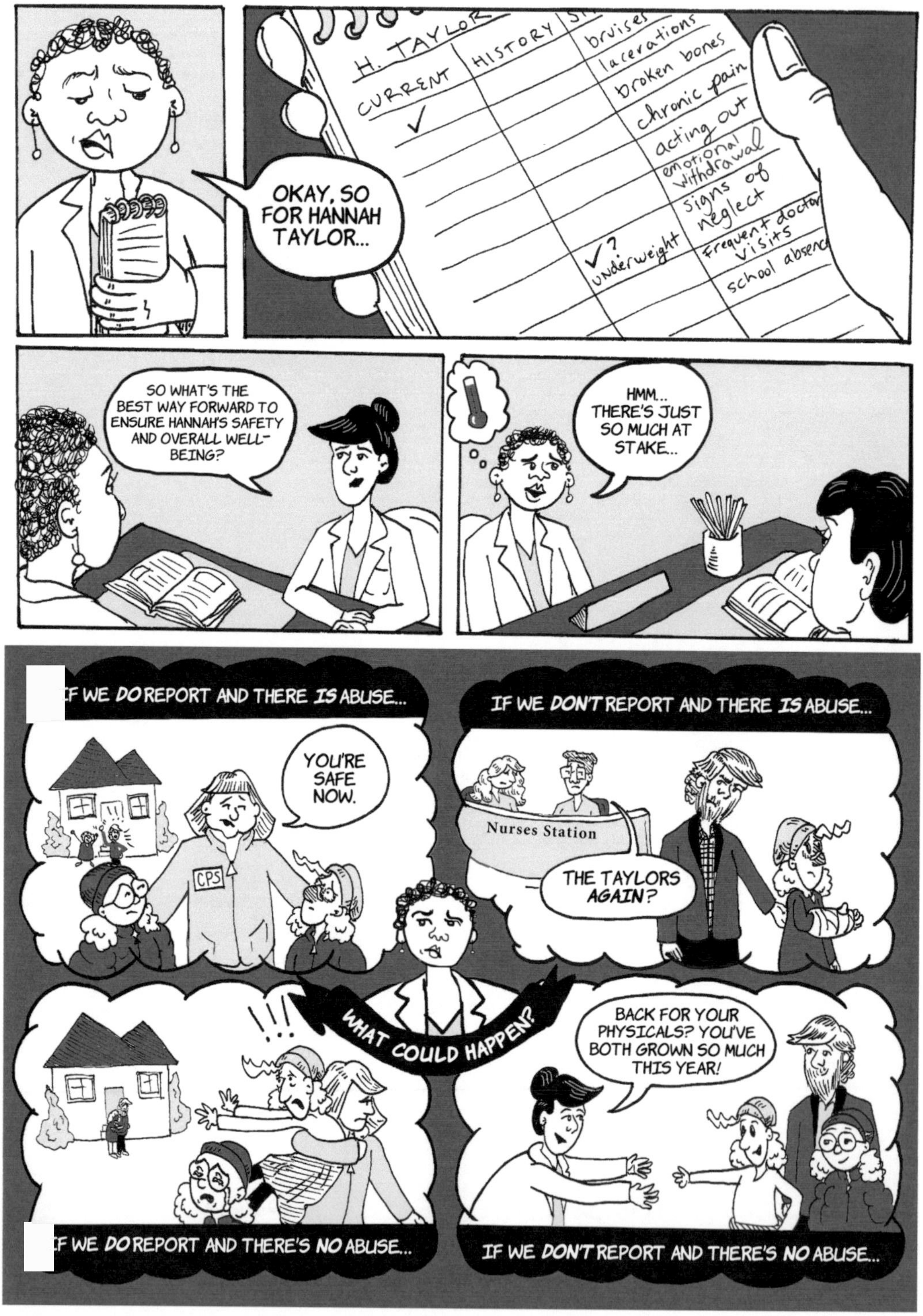
H. TAYLOR
CURRENT
HISTORY
✓
bruises
lacerations
broken bones
chronic pain
acting out
emotional withdrawal
signs of neglect
✓? underweight
frequent docto
visits
school absenc
OKAY, SO FOR HANNAH TAYLOR...
SO WHAT'S THE BEST WAY FORWARD TO ENSURE HANNAH'S SAFETY AND OVERALL WELL-BEING?
HMM... THERE'S JUST SO MUCH AT STAKE...
F WE DO REPORT AND THERE IS ABUSE...
YOU'RE SAFE NOW.
CPS
IF WE DON'T REPORT AND THERE IS ABUSE...
Nurses Station
THE TAYLORS AGAIN?
WHAT COULD HAPPEN?
!!!
BACK FOR YOUR PHYSICALS? YOU'VE BOTH GROWN SO MUCH THIS YEAR!
F WE DO REPORT AND THERE'S NO ABUSE...
IF WE DON'T REPORT AND THERE'S NO ABUSE...

Discussion

Vulnerable populations—children, the elderly, domestic partners, and those with certain kinds of disabilities (e.g., cognitive impairment)—are susceptible to mistreatment by those who are responsible for their physical and emotional well-being. Physical and psychological injuries come in many forms, including bodily wounds, neglect (intentional or unintentional), financial exploitation, and abandonment. Medical professionals are mandated reporters of suspected abuse, as are school employees, religious leaders, and indeed any individual responsible for the welfare of a vulnerable person by virtue of the individual's role in that person's routine activities—for instance, a paid caregiver or a nursing home volunteer. In short, any individual who is an essential part of any program or service provided to the vulnerable person must report suspected abuse of that person.

The case of the Taylor family originates with my (KM) colleague, Dr. Benjamin H. Levi, a medical ethicist and pediatrician who generously gave us permission to render this story in comic form. Dr. Levi and Professor Sharon G. Portwood posit this case in their coauthored article titled "Reasonable Suspicion of Child Abuse: Finding a Common Language." They point out that "all 50 United States have laws that mandate reporting by anyone whose professional work brings them into routine contact with children . . . [and that] in 18 states *any competent adult* is designated a mandated reporter" when there is reasonable suspicion that a child is being abused (Levi and Portwood 64). It can be challenging to determine what constitutes "reasonable suspicion," though, and to decide whether and when to report suspected abuse. One reason for this difficulty is that the "vast majority of child abuse cases do not involve severe maltreatment, so the signs of abuse are often subtle" (63).

In this comic, because the injury to Hannah's nose has no clear cause, both Miss Melanie and Dr. Blanchard independently consider—and later discuss—the possibility that Hannah is being abused, perhaps by someone in her family. Burns and fractures would be red flags, of course, but such obvious signs are not present. Subtler indications of abuse might include a child's wearing dirty or ill-fitting clothes that are perhaps also inappropriate for the season (possibly to hide wounds), one who flinches when someone attempts to touch him or her in an appropriate way (a hug of greeting, for instance), and one who is excessively watchful, hesitant, anxious, restless, or withdrawn. To complicate matters further, there is no "profile" for an abuser. Child abuse occurs in every community and at all levels of society, although some situations make it more likely—poor economic and social conditions and various kinds of stress, for example (Levi and Portwood 63).

Considering one's own vantage point is also important: How much time have I spent directly observing the potential victim? How well do I know the potential abuser? How well does the explanation of a suspicious injury "fit," and what's my "gut reaction" or intuition (Levi and Portwood 66)? In short, as Levi says in lectures on suspected child abuse, reporting shouldn't require absolute certainty . . . but it also shouldn't be simply that abuse is a possibility. Someone in a position to report suspected abuse should be as informed as possible, soliciting and carefully reviewing others' assessments of the situation in order to strengthen or weaken the decision to report.

Reporting suspected abuse will fundamentally alter the relationship of the doctor to the patient and the family, and the impact of this change is not without significant consequences. For example, the doctor may be separated from the child completely, which would mean that a trusted, responsible contact—someone to provide safe care, someone to talk to—is no longer available when the child needs somebody the most. As Levi and Portwood indicate, "being reported and/or investigated for child abuse can damage individuals as well as families" (64), particularly if the reporting is in error. Also, "indiscriminate reporting . . . diminishes the effectiveness of child protection services by dispersing already scarce resources, and eroding confidence in the system" (65). These tensions complicate and may even cloud decision-making as one carries out a fundamental responsibility to protect the child.

Questions for Further Reflection

1. Consider the appearance of the characters—their facial expressions, body language, and actions. How do these aspects of the comic impact your own assessment of potential risk to Hannah and to Sarah?

2. Compare Dr. Blanchard's and Miss Melanie's suspicions. When does each of them begin to suspect potential abuse, and what is the reasoning process that each uses to decide whether or not to report?

3. Consider how Dr. Blanchard responds to Mr. Taylor's anger when he thinks that she is insinuating child abuse. To what extent—and how—are Dr. Blanchard's statements effective in terms of obtaining the X-rays and maintaining trust with Hannah and her father?

4. See the large panel at the end of the comic and think through each of the four scenarios in terms of the impact on Hannah, Sarah, their father, their mother, Dr. Blanchard, Miss Melanie, and Child Protective Services (or "the system").

5. What decision would you make in this situation? Why?

6. Discuss "suspicion" in this comic. Who is suspicious of whom and in what ways? How does suspicion impact each character's responses to the other characters?

7. How does the symbol of a thermometer function in the comic? What are some other visual metaphors that might be equally appropriate?

Related Readings

Carver, Raymond. "Little Things." *Where I'm Calling From: New and Selected Stories,* Random House, 1989.

Levi, Benjamin H., and Sharon G. Portwood. "Reasonable Suspicion of Child Abuse: Finding a Common Language." *Journal of Law, Medicine and Ethics,* Spring 2011, pp. 62–69.

Roethke, Theodore. "My Papa's Waltz." *Collected Poems of Theodore Roethke,* Doubleday, 1937.

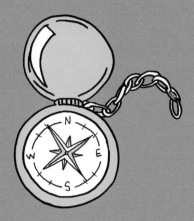

Chapter 5

Confidentiality

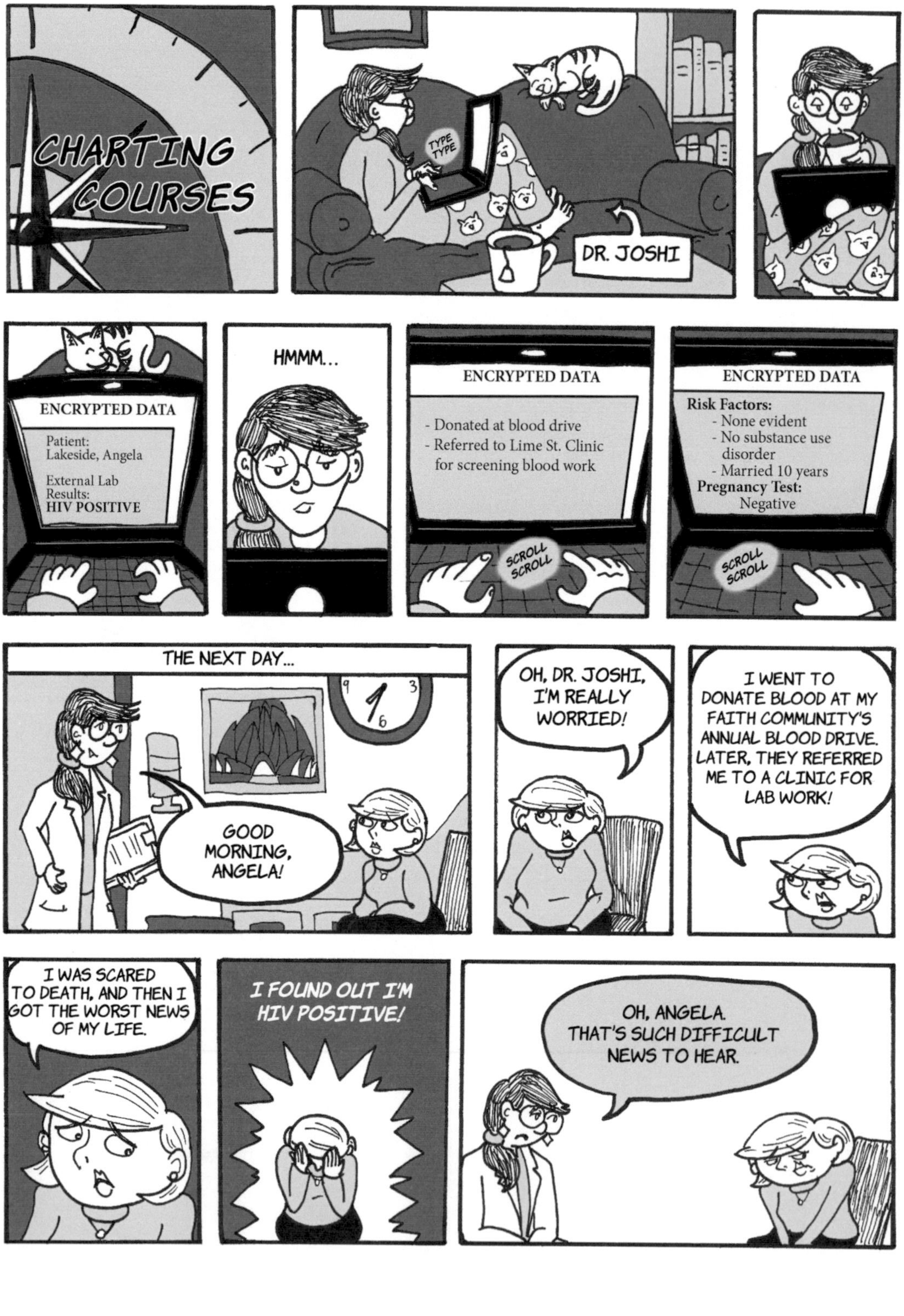
CHARTING COURSES
TYPE TYPE
DR. JOSHI
ENCRYPTED DATA
Patient: Lakeside, Angela
External Lab Results: HIV POSITIVE
HMMM...
ENCRYPTED DATA
- Donated at blood drive
- Referred to Lime St. Clinic for screening blood work
SCROLL SCROLL
ENCRYPTED DATA
Risk Factors:
- None evident
- No substance use disorder
- Married 10 years
Pregnancy Test: Negative
SCROLL SCROLL
THE NEXT DAY...
GOOD MORNING, ANGELA!
OH, DR. JOSHI, I'M REALLY WORRIED!
I WENT TO DONATE BLOOD AT MY FAITH COMMUNITY'S ANNUAL BLOOD DRIVE. LATER, THEY REFERRED ME TO A CLINIC FOR LAB WORK!
I WAS SCARED TO DEATH, AND THEN I GOT THE WORST NEWS OF MY LIFE.
I FOUND OUT I'M HIV POSITIVE!
OH, ANGELA. THAT'S SUCH DIFFICULT NEWS TO HEAR.

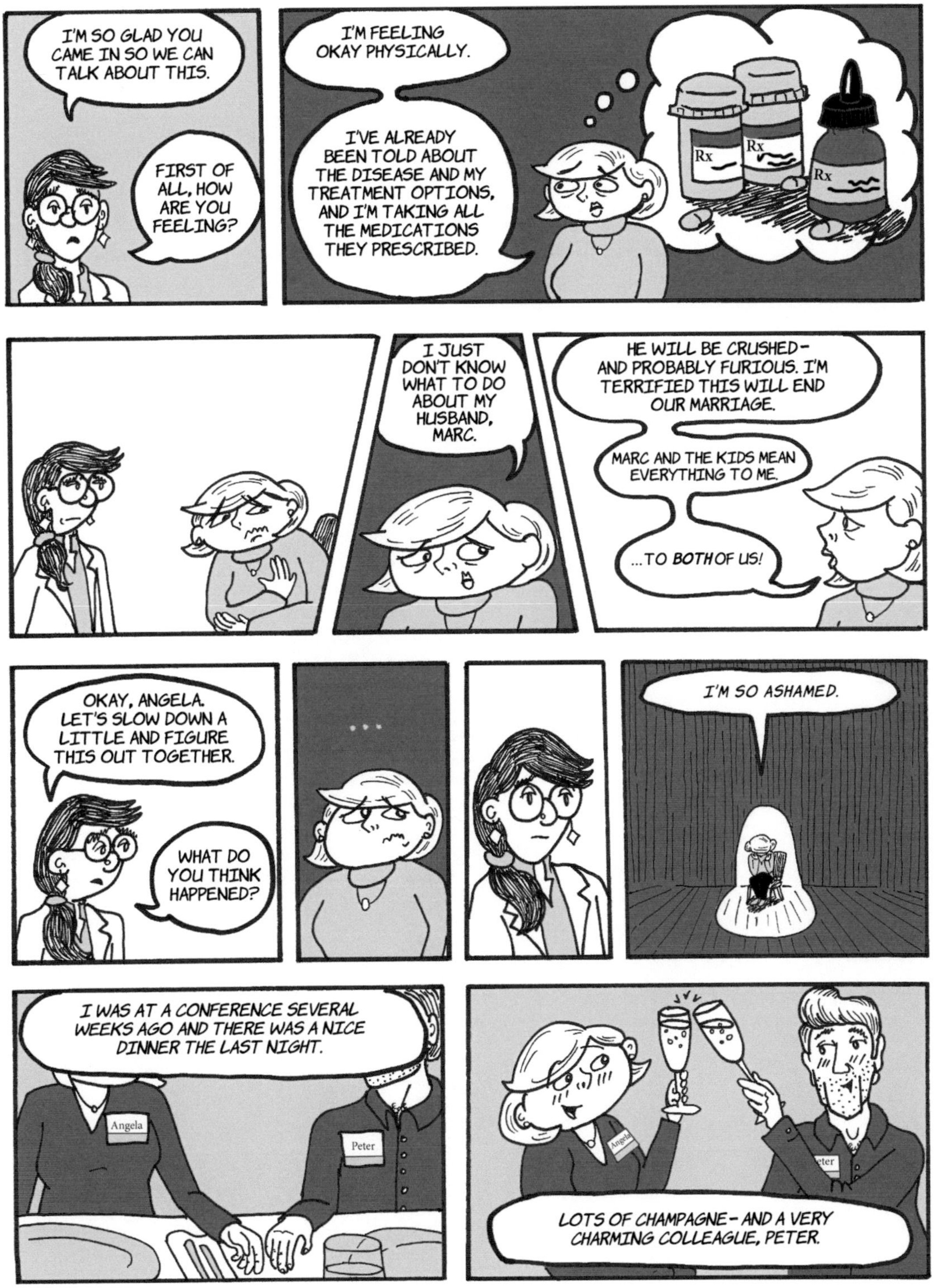
I'M SO GLAD YOU CAME IN SO WE CAN TALK ABOUT THIS.
FIRST OF ALL, HOW ARE YOU FEELING?
I'M FEELING OKAY PHYSICALLY.
I'VE ALREADY BEEN TOLD ABOUT THE DISEASE AND MY TREATMENT OPTIONS, AND I'M TAKING ALL THE MEDICATIONS THEY PRESCRIBED.
Rx
Rx
Rx
I JUST DON'T KNOW WHAT TO DO ABOUT MY HUSBAND, MARC.
HE WILL BE CRUSHED–AND PROBABLY FURIOUS. I'M TERRIFIED THIS WILL END OUR MARRIAGE.
MARC AND THE KIDS MEAN EVERYTHING TO ME.
...TO *BOTH* OF US!
OKAY, ANGELA. LET'S SLOW DOWN A LITTLE AND FIGURE THIS OUT TOGETHER.
WHAT DO YOU THINK HAPPENED?
...
I'M SO ASHAMED.
I WAS AT A CONFERENCE SEVERAL WEEKS AGO AND THERE WAS A NICE DINNER THE LAST NIGHT.
Angela
Peter
LOTS OF CHAMPAGNE–AND A VERY CHARMING COLLEAGUE, PETER.

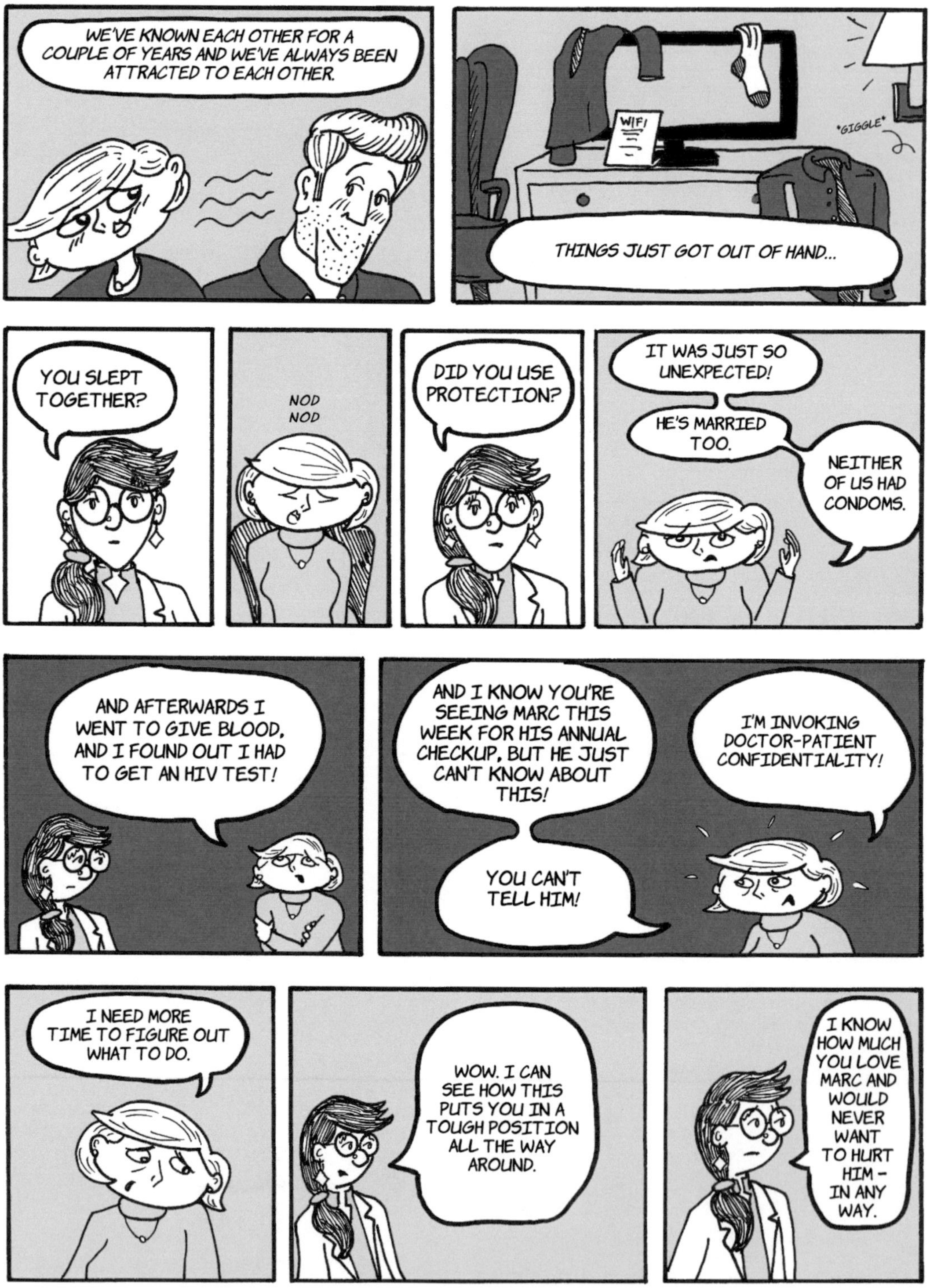
WE'VE KNOWN EACH OTHER FOR A COUPLE OF YEARS AND WE'VE ALWAYS BEEN ATTRACTED TO EACH OTHER.
WIFI
GIGGLE
THINGS JUST GOT OUT OF HAND...
YOU SLEPT TOGETHER?
NOD NOD
DID YOU USE PROTECTION?
IT WAS JUST SO UNEXPECTED!
HE'S MARRIED TOO.
NEITHER OF US HAD CONDOMS.
AND AFTERWARDS I WENT TO GIVE BLOOD, AND I FOUND OUT I HAD TO GET AN HIV TEST!
AND I KNOW YOU'RE SEEING MARC THIS WEEK FOR HIS ANNUAL CHECKUP, BUT HE JUST CAN'T KNOW ABOUT THIS!
YOU CAN'T TELL HIM!
I'M INVOKING DOCTOR-PATIENT CONFIDENTIALITY!
I NEED MORE TIME TO FIGURE OUT WHAT TO DO.
WOW. I CAN SEE HOW THIS PUTS YOU IN A TOUGH POSITION ALL THE WAY AROUND.
I KNOW HOW MUCH YOU LOVE MARC AND WOULD NEVER WANT TO HURT HIM — IN ANY WAY.

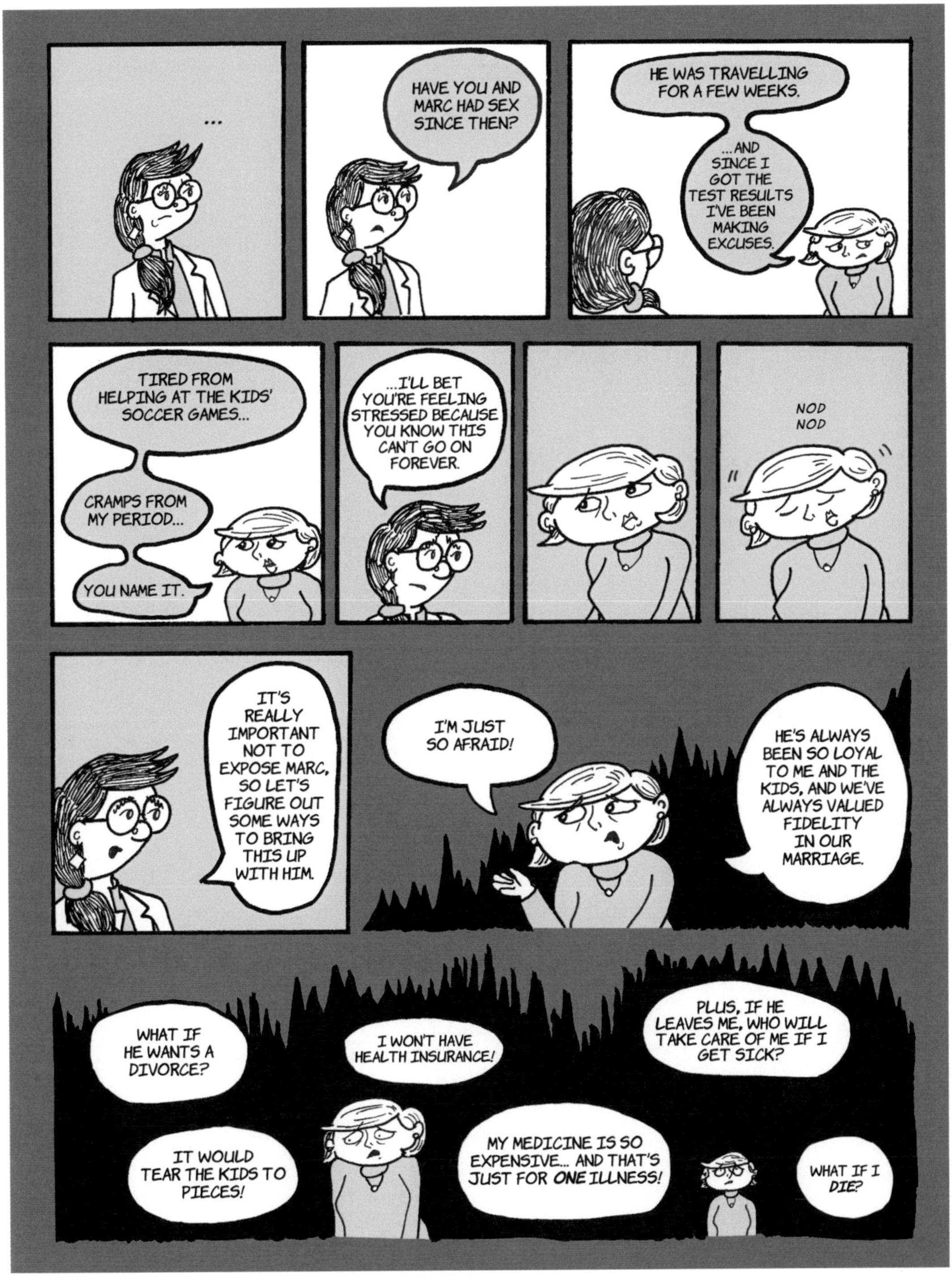
...
HAVE YOU AND MARC HAD SEX SINCE THEN?
HE WAS TRAVELLING FOR A FEW WEEKS.
...AND SINCE I GOT THE TEST RESULTS I'VE BEEN MAKING EXCUSES.
TIRED FROM HELPING AT THE KIDS' SOCCER GAMES...
CRAMPS FROM MY PERIOD...
YOU NAME IT.
...I'LL BET YOU'RE FEELING STRESSED BECAUSE YOU KNOW THIS CAN'T GO ON FOREVER.
NOD NOD
IT'S REALLY IMPORTANT NOT TO EXPOSE MARC, SO LET'S FIGURE OUT SOME WAYS TO BRING THIS UP WITH HIM.
I'M JUST SO AFRAID!
HE'S ALWAYS BEEN SO LOYAL TO ME AND THE KIDS, AND WE'VE ALWAYS VALUED FIDELITY IN OUR MARRIAGE.
WHAT IF HE WANTS A DIVORCE?
I WON'T HAVE HEALTH INSURANCE!
PLUS, IF HE LEAVES ME, WHO WILL TAKE CARE OF ME IF I GET SICK?
IT WOULD TEAR THE KIDS TO PIECES!
MY MEDICINE IS SO EXPENSIVE... AND THAT'S JUST FOR ONE ILLNESS!
WHAT IF I DIE?

SOB
CRY
SOB
SO PLEASE DON'T TELL HIM!
LET'S TAKE A STEP BACK TO SEE IF WE CAN BALANCE YOUR NEEDS WITH MARC'S.
OKAY
I KNOW YOUR STRONG MORAL COMPASS, AND I KNOW YOU'LL WANT TO DO ALL YOU CAN TO DO RIGHT BY MARC.
N
MY FAMILY IS THE MOST IMPORTANT THING IN MY LIFE ...
WHERE DO I GO FROM HERE?

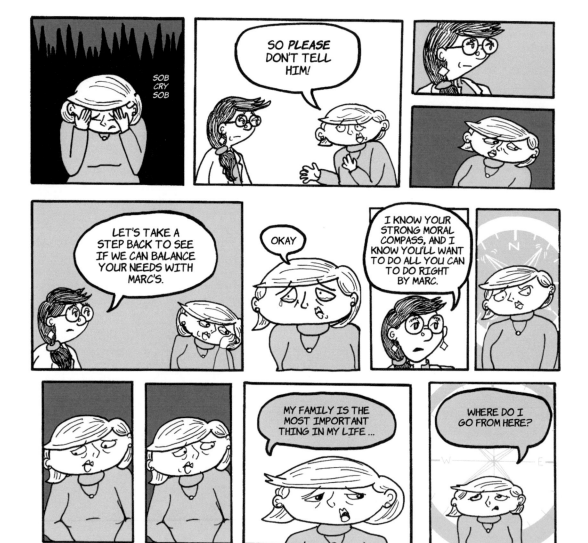

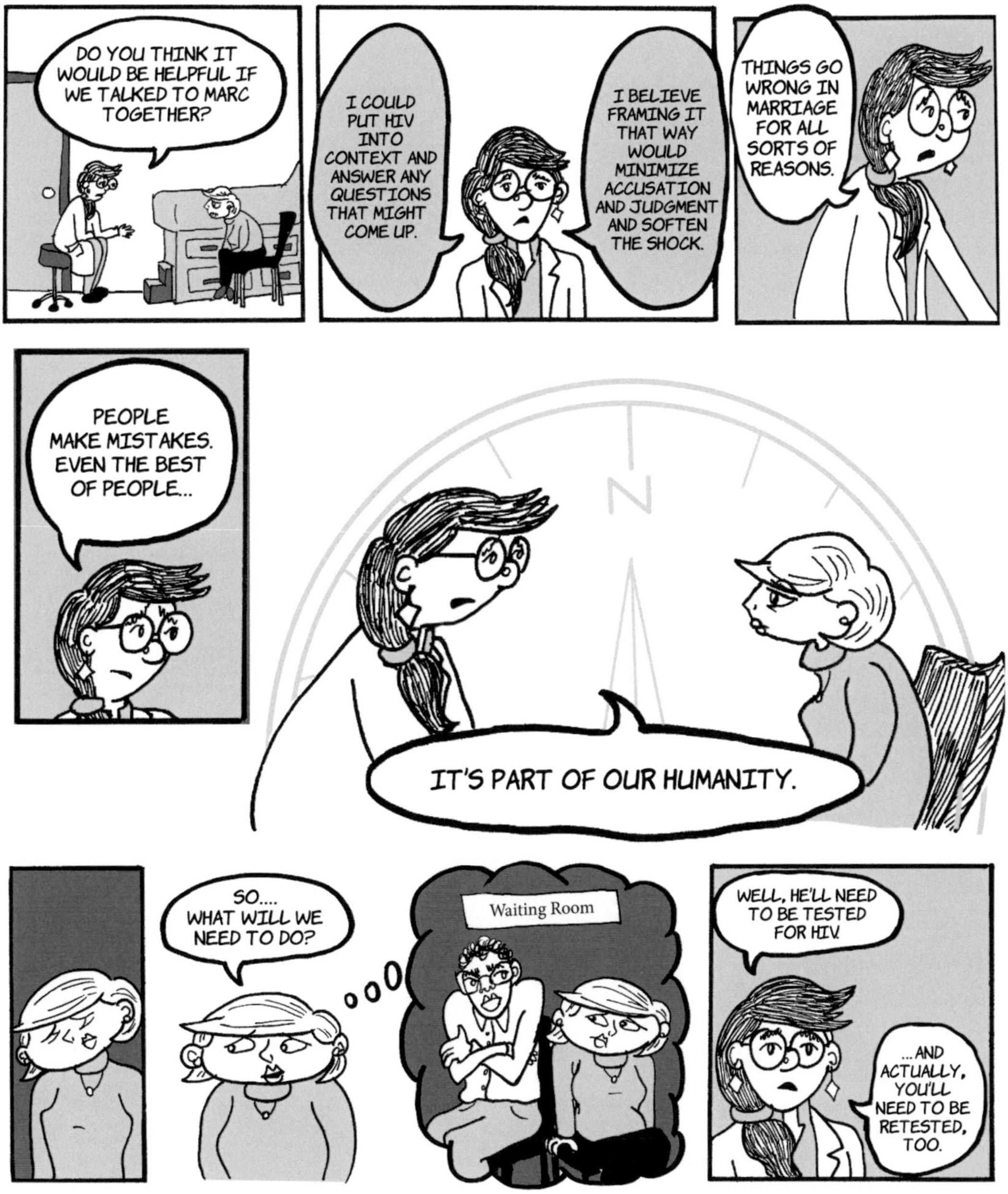
DO YOU THINK IT WOULD BE HELPFUL IF WE TALKED TO MARC TOGETHER?
I COULD PUT HIV INTO CONTEXT AND ANSWER ANY QUESTIONS THAT MIGHT COME UP.
I BELIEVE FRAMING IT THAT WAY WOULD MINIMIZE ACCUSATION AND JUDGMENT AND SOFTEN THE SHOCK.
THINGS GO WRONG IN MARRIAGE FOR ALL SORTS OF REASONS.
PEOPLE MAKE MISTAKES. EVEN THE BEST OF PEOPLE...
N
IT'S PART OF OUR HUMANITY.
SO.... WHAT WILL WE NEED TO DO?
Waiting Room
WELL, HE'LL NEED TO BE TESTED FOR HIV.
...AND ACTUALLY, YOU'LL NEED TO BE RETESTED, TOO.

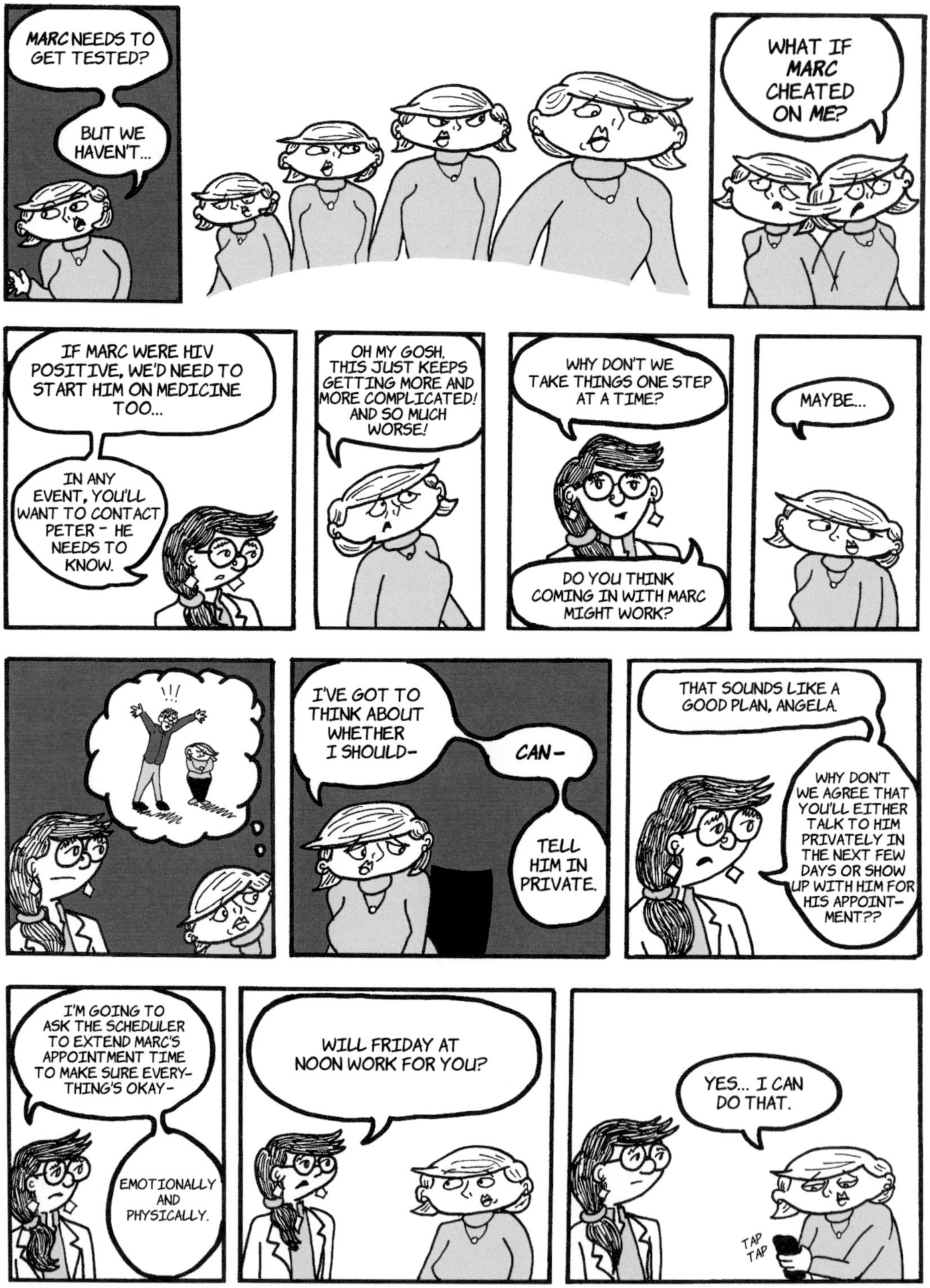
MARC NEEDS TO GET TESTED?
BUT WE HAVEN'T...
WHAT IF MARC CHEATED ON ME?
IF MARC WERE HIV POSITIVE, WE'D NEED TO START HIM ON MEDICINE TOO...
IN ANY EVENT, YOU'LL WANT TO CONTACT PETER - HE NEEDS TO KNOW.
OH MY GOSH, THIS JUST KEEPS GETTING MORE AND MORE COMPLICATED! AND SO MUCH WORSE!
WHY DON'T WE TAKE THINGS ONE STEP AT A TIME?
DO YOU THINK COMING IN WITH MARC MIGHT WORK?
MAYBE...
!!!
I'VE GOT TO THINK ABOUT WHETHER I SHOULD-
CAN-
TELL HIM IN PRIVATE.
THAT SOUNDS LIKE A GOOD PLAN, ANGELA.
WHY DON'T WE AGREE THAT YOU'LL EITHER TALK TO HIM PRIVATELY IN THE NEXT FEW DAYS OR SHOW UP WITH HIM FOR HIS APPOINT-MENT??
I'M GOING TO ASK THE SCHEDULER TO EXTEND MARC'S APPOINTMENT TIME TO MAKE SURE EVERY-THING'S OKAY-
EMOTIONALLY AND PHYSICALLY.
WILL FRIDAY AT NOON WORK FOR YOU?
YES... I CAN DO THAT.
TAP TAP

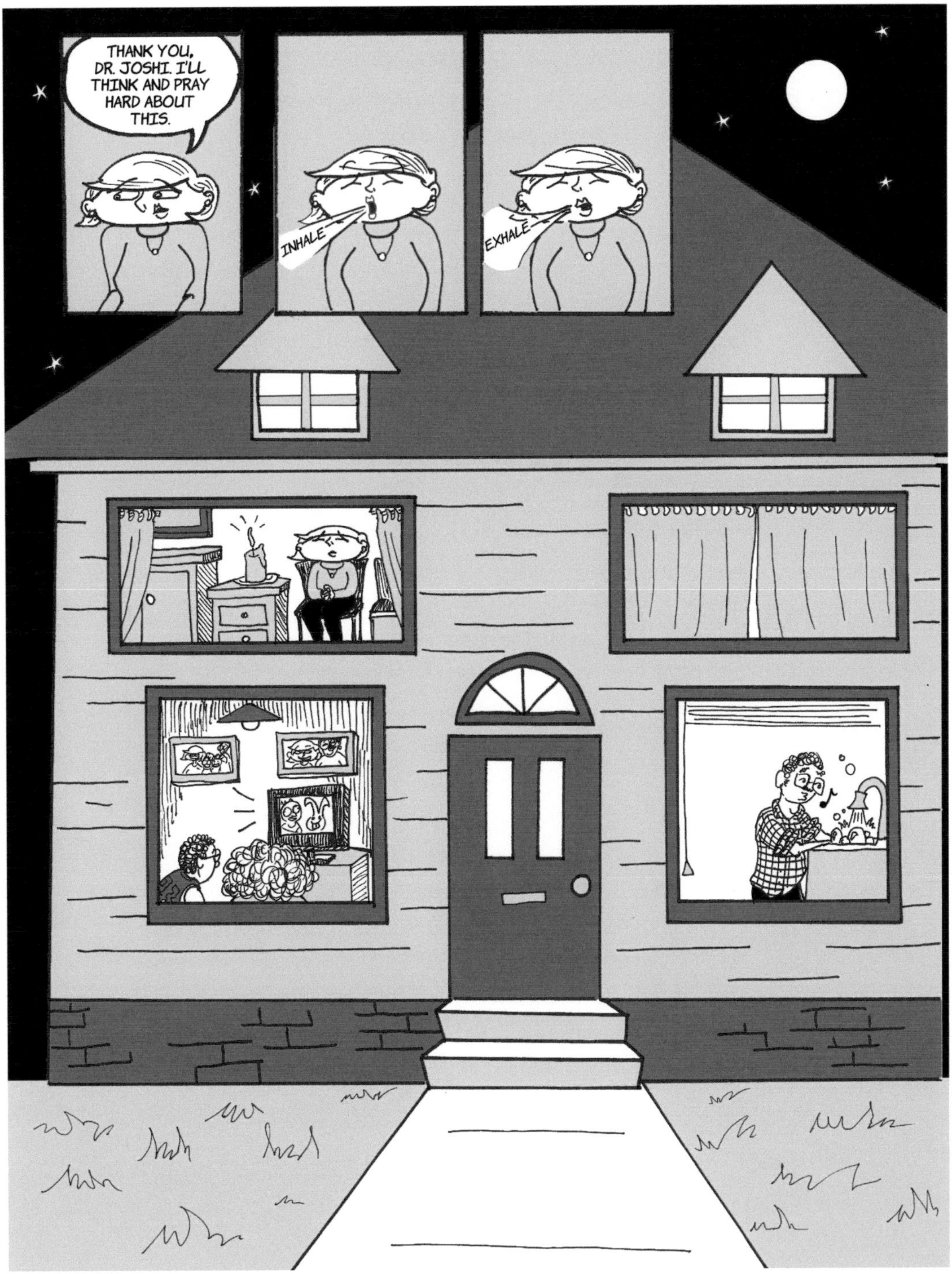
THANK YOU, DR. JOSHI. I'LL THINK AND PRAY HARD ABOUT THIS.
INHALE
EXHALE

Discussion

To provide effective medical care, physicians must be comfortable discussing physical conditions and associated psychosocial issues such as sexual history and substance use. And in order to be comfortable sharing such private information, patients must feel safe with their providers; they must have confidence that intimate details will remain confidential. Confidentiality is at the heart of the doctor-patient relationship. It is necessary for the kind of trust that contributes to overall well-being. When a provider earns a patient's trust, a fruitful and even warm partnership can evolve. But when a patient's confidentiality is violated, the patient can lose trust in the physician and might therefore withhold sensitive information that would be vital to diagnosis and even prognosis.

Respecting confidentiality sounds relatively simple: just don't share information with those who do not have a right to such knowledge, and don't access information (via an electronic medical record, for instance) without a legitimate need to know. As is evident in this comic, however, issues of confidentiality can be complex, and, as Angela imagines, the consequences of a breach in confidentiality can be devastating.

In *Charting Courses*, confidentiality is complicated by Dr. Joshi's conflict of obligation. Because she is also the physician for Angela's husband, Marc, Dr. Joshi has a fiduciary responsibility to ensure his physical well-being and preserve the (presumed) trust inherent in their own doctor-patient relationship. To honor Angela's request for complete confidentiality is to dishonor Marc's interest in knowing about his risk for contracting HIV. In the absence of this knowledge, Marc cannot exercise autonomy; he cannot determine what to do with regard to his and Angela's sexual intimacy in order to protect himself from disease. Dr. Joshi's quandary signals the way that ethical—and sometimes legal—responsibilities can conflict on a larger scale as well. Consider, for example, how two topics that feature prominently in clinical ethics teaching and practice might seem at odds: the Health Information Portability and Accountability Act of 1996 (HIPAA), which guides U.S. law regarding the privacy of an individual's medical information, and the Tarasoff Rule (codified in 1985), which holds that "protective privilege ends where public peril begins." So what are the limits of confidentiality?

The following are legitimate reasons to breach confidentiality in order to protect third parties from harm: contagious diseases (e.g., COVID-19, HIV, tuberculosis), impaired driving/cognition (e.g., from seizure disorders, from dementia), abuse and neglect of vulnerable persons or an explicit threat to a specific person (e.g., children, elders, domestic partners), and violent crimes (e.g., knife and gunshot wounds). Even as healthcare providers have a duty to protect the public good in these situations, however, only minimal information about the patient should be revealed so that the person is shielded from potential personal, social, and economic consequences. These might include psychological trauma and stigma (in the context of domestic abuse or rape, for example) or denial of employment (e.g., in the context of debilitating diseases like cancer). Here, the principle of nonmaleficence—do no harm—is at stake.

In this comic we witness Dr. Joshi in action as she balances the needs of multiple stakeholders. While we are not told the ultimate outcome, she has preserved the trust and support that she and Angela have developed over the course of their professional relationship, and that is a big success in its own right.

Questions for Further Reflection

1. Consider the impact and implications of being notified that you have HIV. What are some of the feelings you might have if you received this new diagnosis? What other diagnoses could, if made public, potentially lead to significant social, economic, familial, or other consequences?

2. As authors of this comic, we chose particular traits for the character of Angela that were not in the original case (e.g., socioeconomic status, spiritual orientation). What message(s) might we have been trying to send by making these choices?

3. What does Angela realize in the panels at the top of the next-to-last page, and why is that important to the story?

4. *Charting Courses* has more wordless panels than a typical comic. Why?

5. Consider Dr. Joshi's attitude and behavior during her visit with Angela. What are other ways she might have worked with Angela in this circumstance, and how might those differences have influenced the outcome?

6. If you were Dr. Joshi, what would you do if Angela did not show up with Marc and did not contact you—assuming that Marc did not indicate any misgivings that he might be at risk for HIV?

Note

We thank our colleagues at Drexel University College of Medicine, Dr. Dennis Novack and Dr. Janet Fleetwood, for creating an excellent case (originally known as "HIV and Confidentiality: Susan Lakeside") and for granting us permission to use it as the basis of this comic.

Related Readings

Fleck, Leonard, and Marcia Angell. "Case Study: 'Please Don't Tell!'" *The Social Medicine Reader*, edited by Gail E. Henderson et al., Duke UP, 1997, pp. 349–52.

Halevy, Amir. "Confidentiality." *20 Common Problems: Ethics in Primary Care*, edited by Jeremy Sugarman, McGraw-Hill, 2000, pp. 149–60.

Klass, Perri. "Invasions." *A Not Entirely Benign Procedure*, G. P. Putnam's Sons, 1987, pp. 103–8.

Latner, Ann W. "Social Media Post Prompts Firing." *Clinical Advisor*, 22 May 2019, www.clinicaladvisor.com/home/my-prac tice/legal-advisor/social-media-post -prompts-firing/.

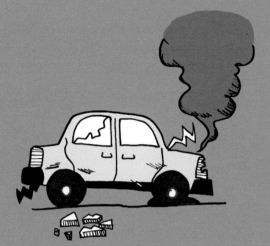

Chapter 6

Medical Mistakes and Truth-Telling

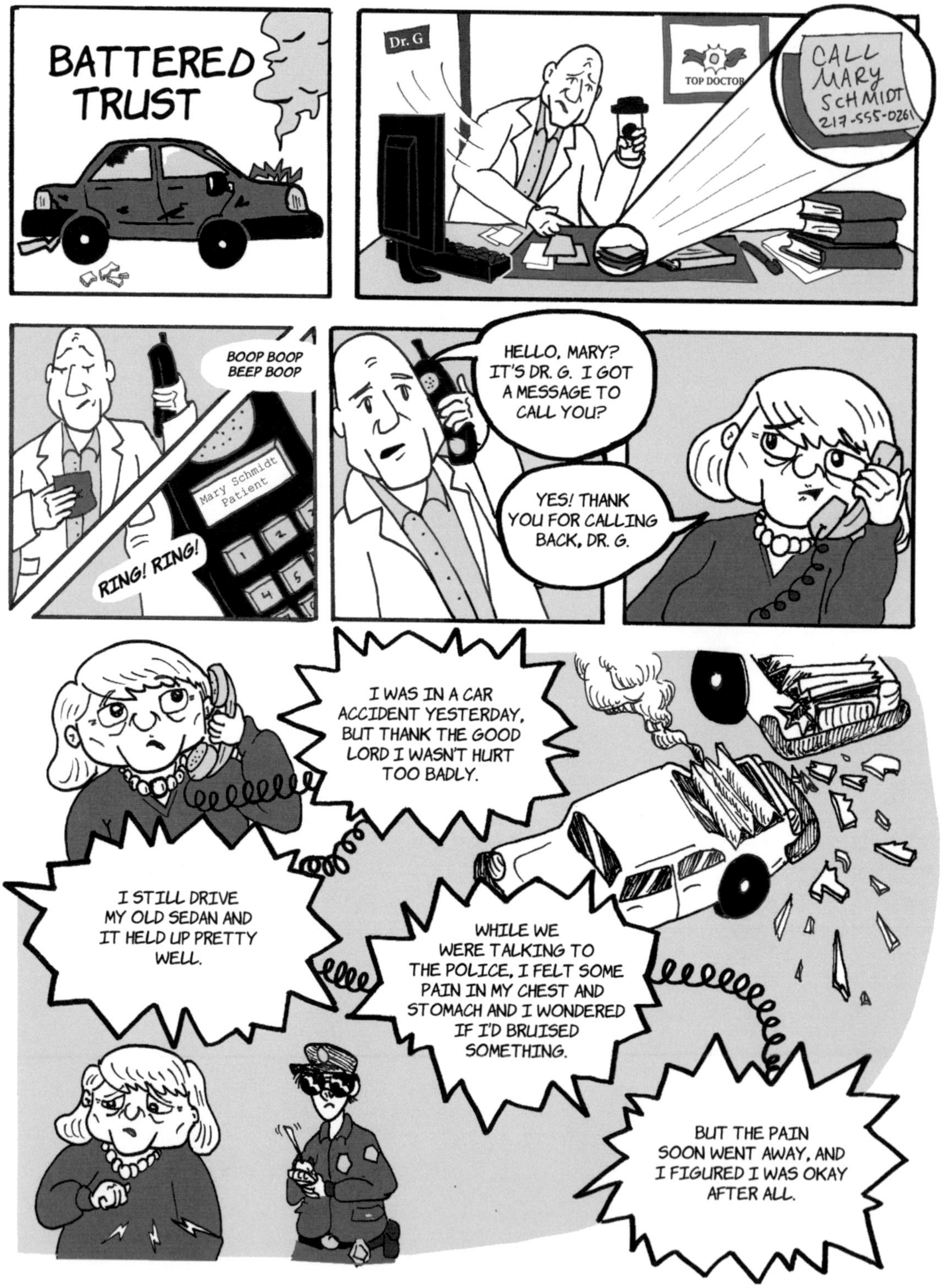
BATTERED TRUST
Dr. G
TOP DOCTOR
CALL MARY SCHMIDT 217-555-0261
BOOP BOOP BEEP BOOP
Mary Schmidt Patient
RING! RING!
HELLO, MARY? IT'S DR. G. I GOT A MESSAGE TO CALL YOU?
YES! THANK YOU FOR CALLING BACK, DR. G.
I WAS IN A CAR ACCIDENT YESTERDAY, BUT THANK THE GOOD LORD I WASN'T HURT TOO BADLY.
I STILL DRIVE MY OLD SEDAN AND IT HELD UP PRETTY WELL.
WHILE WE WERE TALKING TO THE POLICE, I FELT SOME PAIN IN MY CHEST AND STOMACH AND I WONDERED IF I'D BRUISED SOMETHING.
BUT THE PAIN SOON WENT AWAY, AND I FIGURED I WAS OKAY AFTER ALL.

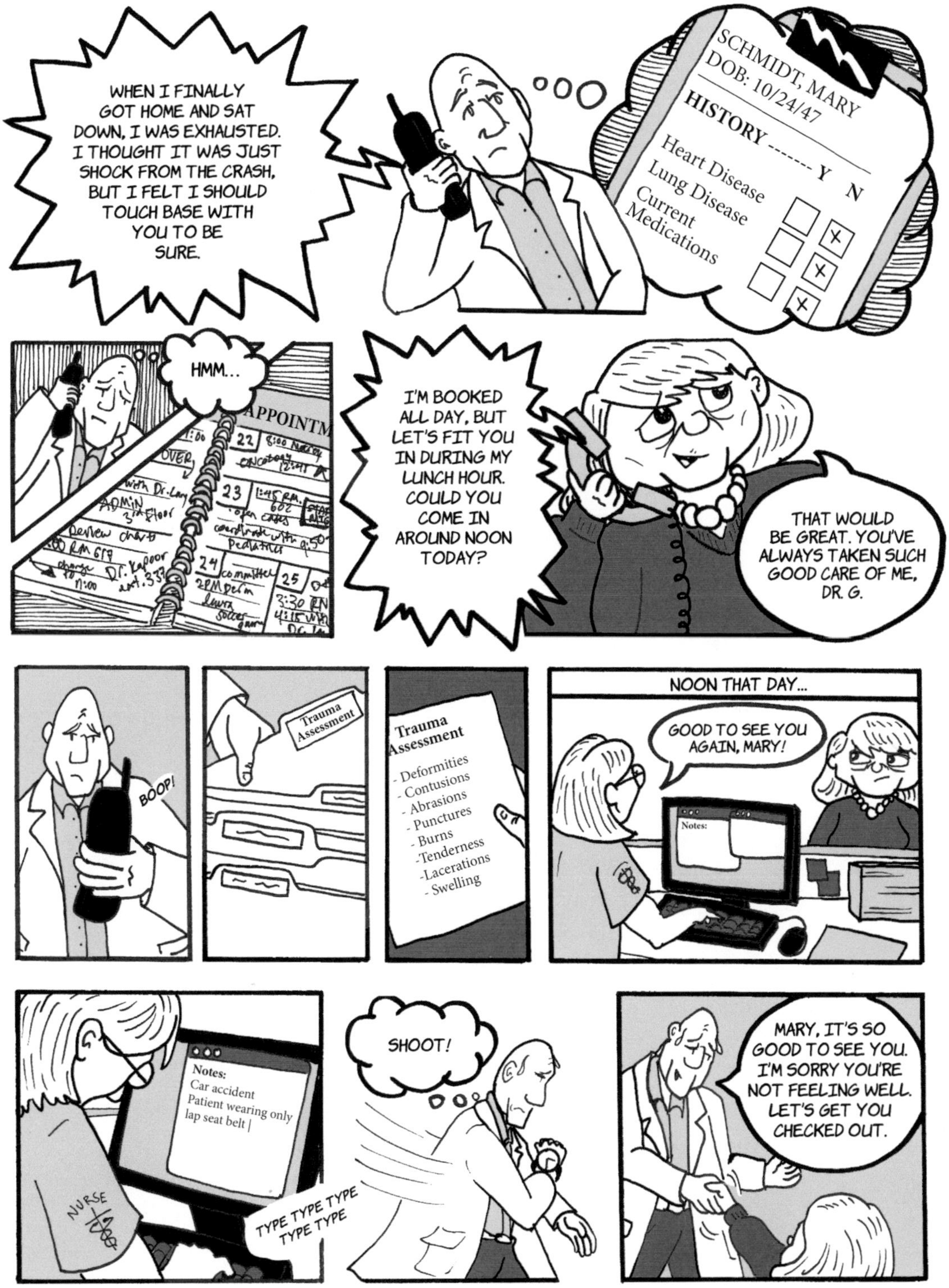
WHEN I FINALLY GOT HOME AND SAT DOWN, I WAS EXHAUSTED. I THOUGHT IT WAS JUST SHOCK FROM THE CRASH, BUT I FELT I SHOULD TOUCH BASE WITH YOU TO BE SURE.
SCHMIDT, MARY
DOB: 10/24/47
HISTORY ------- Y N
Heart Disease
Lung Disease
Current Medications
HMM...
APPOINTM
I'M BOOKED ALL DAY, BUT LET'S FIT YOU IN DURING MY LUNCH HOUR. COULD YOU COME IN AROUND NOON TODAY?
THAT WOULD BE GREAT. YOU'VE ALWAYS TAKEN SUCH GOOD CARE OF ME, DR. G.
BOOP!
Trauma Assessment
Trauma Assessment
- Deformities
- Contusions
- Abrasions
- Punctures
- Burns
-Tenderness
-Lacerations
- Swelling
NOON THAT DAY...
GOOD TO SEE YOU AGAIN, MARY!
Notes:
Notes:
Car accident
Patient wearing only lap seat belt |
NURSE
TYPE TYPE TYPE TYPE TYPE
SHOOT!
MARY, IT'S SO GOOD TO SEE YOU. I'M SORRY YOU'RE NOT FEELING WELL. LET'S GET YOU CHECKED OUT.

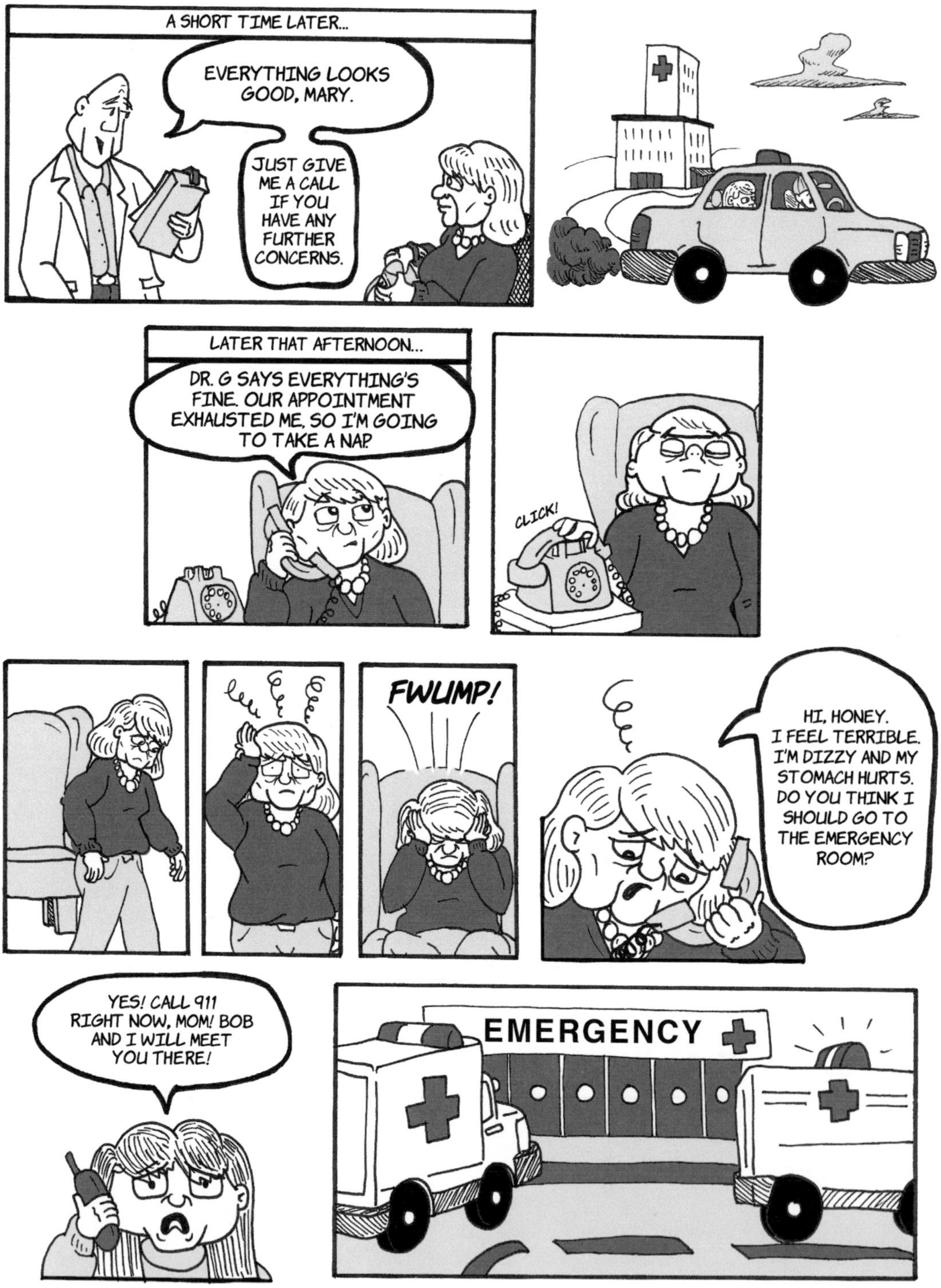
A SHORT TIME LATER...
EVERYTHING LOOKS GOOD, MARY.
JUST GIVE ME A CALL IF YOU HAVE ANY FURTHER CONCERNS.
LATER THAT AFTERNOON...
DR. G SAYS EVERYTHING'S FINE. OUR APPOINTMENT EXHAUSTED ME, SO I'M GOING TO TAKE A NAP.
CLICK!
FWUMP!
HI, HONEY. I FEEL TERRIBLE. I'M DIZZY AND MY STOMACH HURTS. DO YOU THINK I SHOULD GO TO THE EMERGENCY ROOM?
YES! CALL 911 RIGHT NOW, MOM! BOB AND I WILL MEET YOU THERE!
EMERGENCY

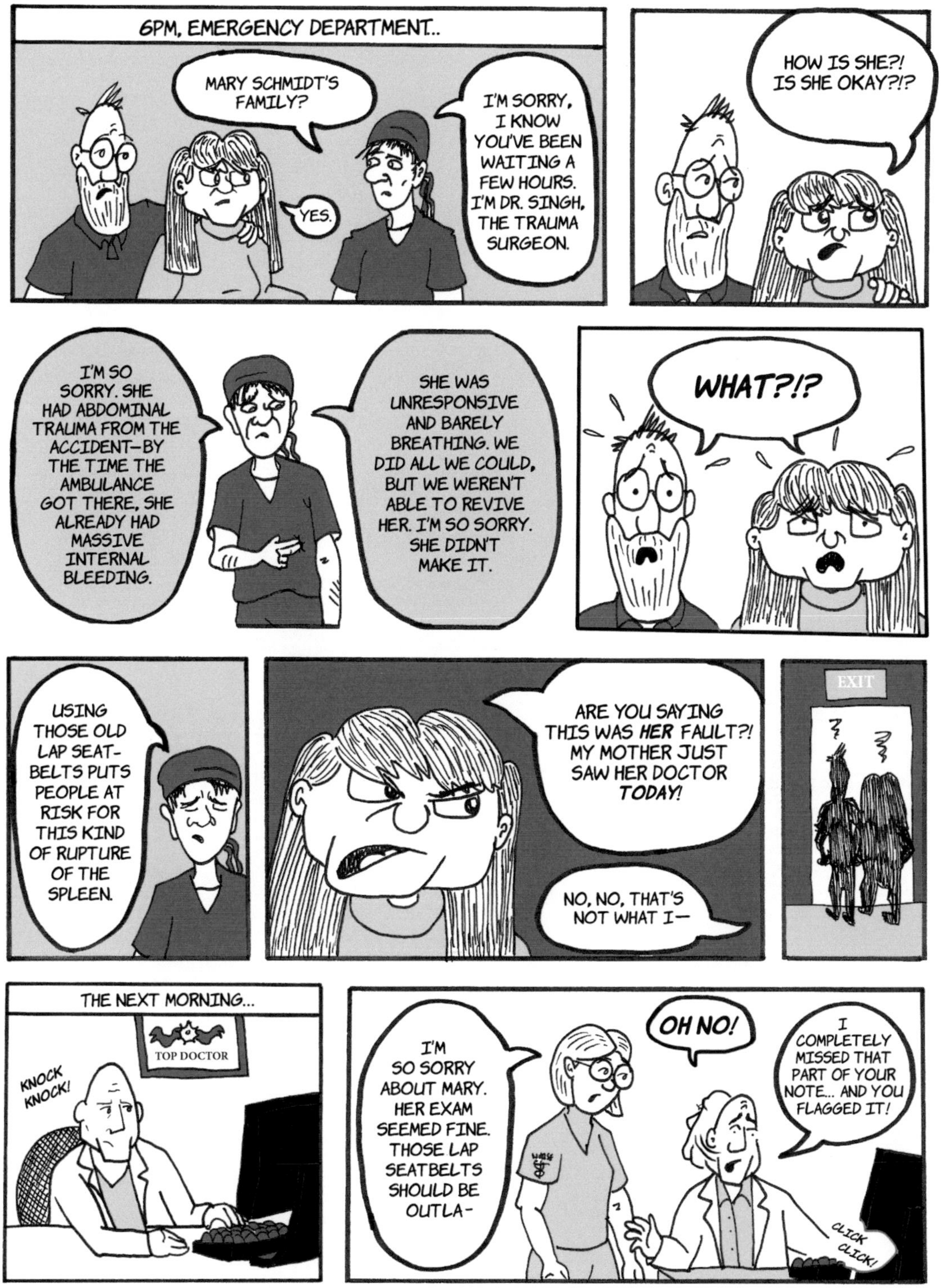
6PM, EMERGENCY DEPARTMENT..
MARY SCHMIDT'S FAMILY?
YES.
I'M SORRY, I KNOW YOU'VE BEEN WAITING A FEW HOURS. I'M DR. SINGH, THE TRAUMA SURGEON.
HOW IS SHE?! IS SHE OKAY?!?
I'M SO SORRY. SHE HAD ABDOMINAL TRAUMA FROM THE ACCIDENT—BY THE TIME THE AMBULANCE GOT THERE, SHE ALREADY HAD MASSIVE INTERNAL BLEEDING.
SHE WAS UNRESPONSIVE AND BARELY BREATHING. WE DID ALL WE COULD, BUT WE WEREN'T ABLE TO REVIVE HER. I'M SO SORRY. SHE DIDN'T MAKE IT.
WHAT?!?
USING THOSE OLD LAP SEAT-BELTS PUTS PEOPLE AT RISK FOR THIS KIND OF RUPTURE OF THE SPLEEN.
ARE YOU SAYING THIS WAS HER FAULT?! MY MOTHER JUST SAW HER DOCTOR TODAY!
NO, NO, THAT'S NOT WHAT I—
EXIT
THE NEXT MORNING...
TOP DOCTOR
KNOCK KNOCK!
I'M SO SORRY ABOUT MARY. HER EXAM SEEMED FINE. THOSE LAP SEATBELTS SHOULD BE OUTLA-
OH NO!
I COMPLETELY MISSED THAT PART OF YOUR NOTE... AND YOU FLAGGED IT!
CLICK CLICK!

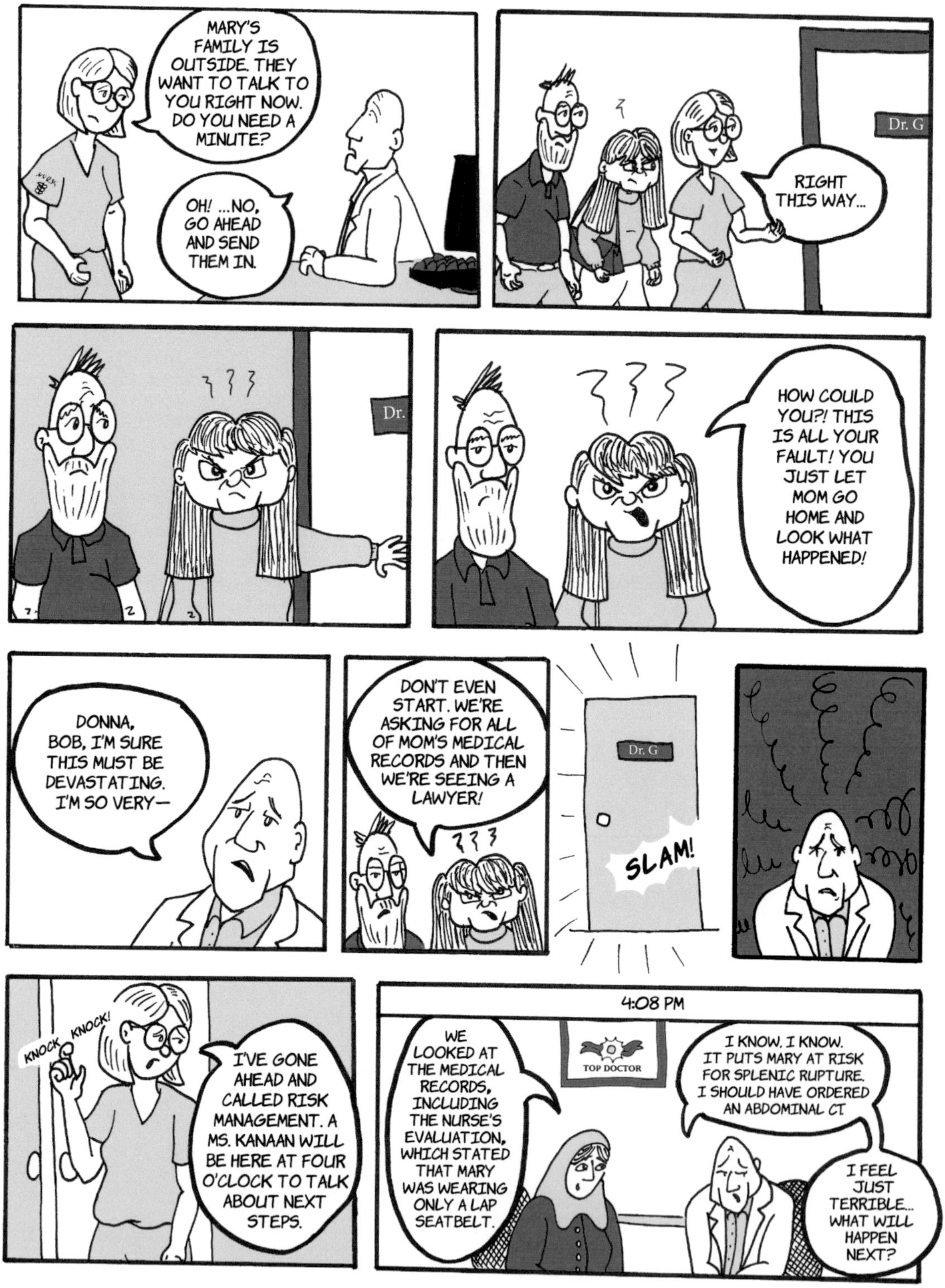
MARY'S FAMILY IS OUTSIDE. THEY WANT TO TALK TO YOU RIGHT NOW. DO YOU NEED A MINUTE?
OH! ...NO, GO AHEAD AND SEND THEM IN.
Dr. G
RIGHT THIS WAY...
Dr.
HOW COULD YOU?! THIS IS ALL YOUR FAULT! YOU JUST LET MOM GO HOME AND LOOK WHAT HAPPENED!
DONNA, BOB, I'M SURE THIS MUST BE DEVASTATING. I'M SO VERY—
DON'T EVEN START. WE'RE ASKING FOR ALL OF MOM'S MEDICAL RECORDS AND THEN WE'RE SEEING A LAWYER!
Dr. G
SLAM!
KNOCK KNOCK!
I'VE GONE AHEAD AND CALLED RISK MANAGEMENT. A MS. KANAAN WILL BE HERE AT FOUR O'CLOCK TO TALK ABOUT NEXT STEPS.
4:08 PM
TOP DOCTOR
WE LOOKED AT THE MEDICAL RECORDS, INCLUDING THE NURSE'S EVALUATION, WHICH STATED THAT MARY WAS WEARING ONLY A LAP SEATBELT.
I KNOW. I KNOW. IT PUTS MARY AT RISK FOR SPLENIC RUPTURE. I SHOULD HAVE ORDERED AN ABDOMINAL CT.
I FEEL JUST TERRIBLE... WHAT WILL HAPPEN NEXT?

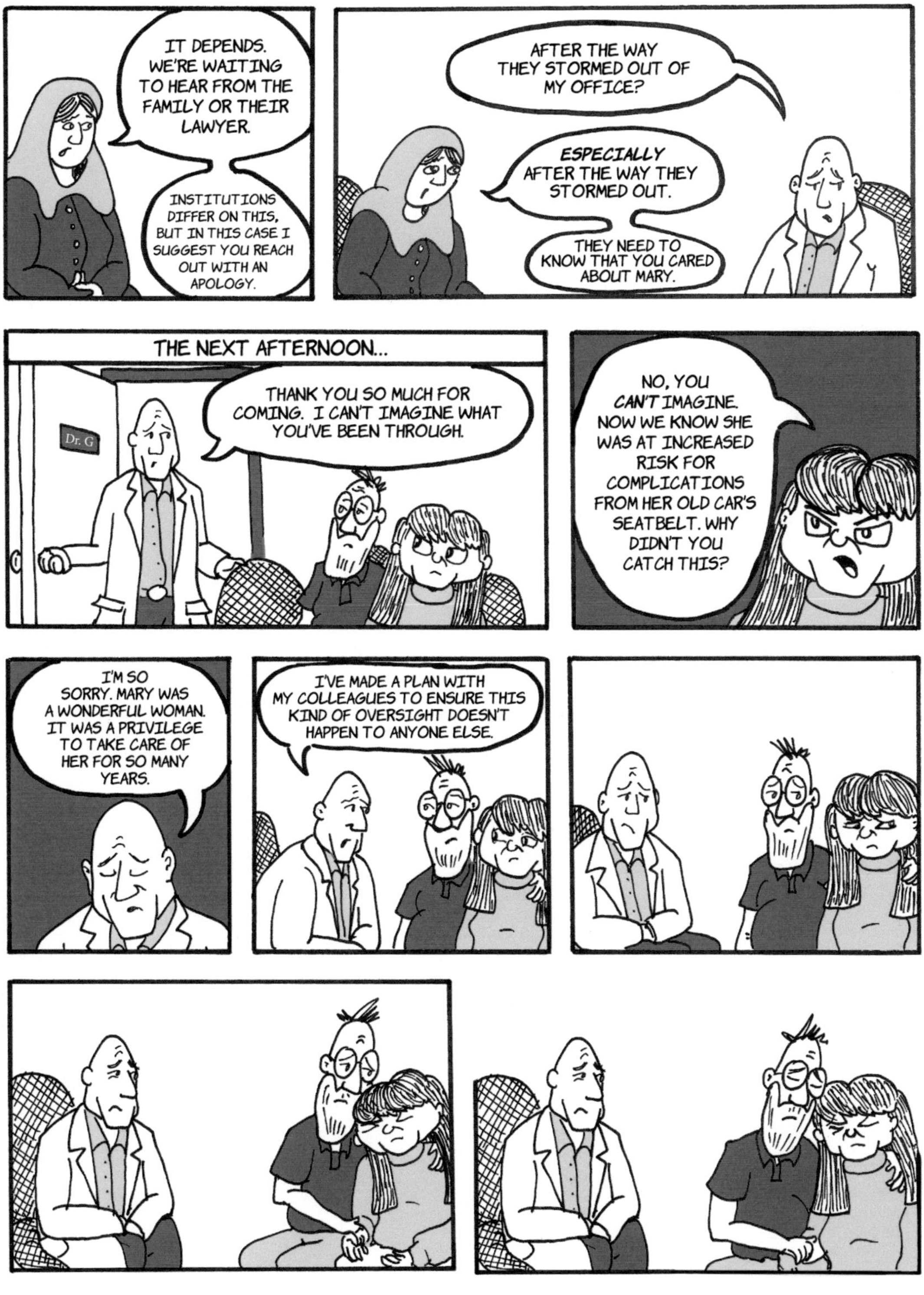
IT DEPENDS. WE'RE WAITING TO HEAR FROM THE FAMILY OR THEIR LAWYER.
INSTITUTIONS DIFFER ON THIS, BUT IN THIS CASE I SUGGEST YOU REACH OUT WITH AN APOLOGY.
AFTER THE WAY THEY STORMED OUT OF MY OFFICE?
ESPECIALLY AFTER THE WAY THEY STORMED OUT.
THEY NEED TO KNOW THAT YOU CARED ABOUT MARY.
THE NEXT AFTERNOON...
Dr. G
THANK YOU SO MUCH FOR COMING. I CAN'T IMAGINE WHAT YOU'VE BEEN THROUGH.
NO, YOU CAN'T IMAGINE. NOW WE KNOW SHE WAS AT INCREASED RISK FOR COMPLICATIONS FROM HER OLD CAR'S SEATBELT. WHY DIDN'T YOU CATCH THIS?
I'M SO SORRY. MARY WAS A WONDERFUL WOMAN. IT WAS A PRIVILEGE TO TAKE CARE OF HER FOR SO MANY YEARS.
I'VE MADE A PLAN WITH MY COLLEAGUES TO ENSURE THIS KIND OF OVERSIGHT DOESN'T HAPPEN TO ANYONE ELSE.

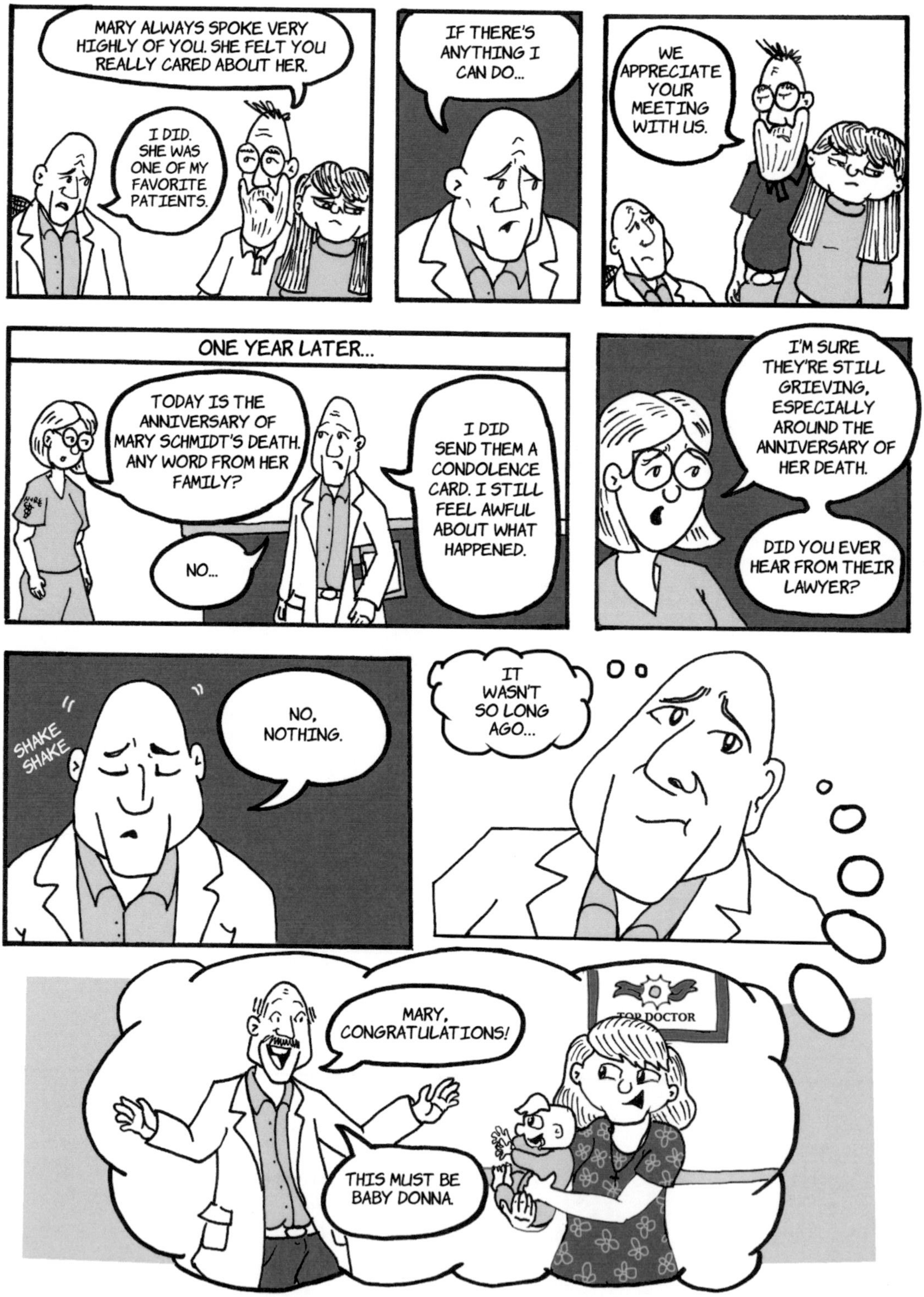
MARY ALWAYS SPOKE VERY HIGHLY OF YOU. SHE FELT YOU REALLY CARED ABOUT HER.
I DID. SHE WAS ONE OF MY FAVORITE PATIENTS.
IF THERE'S ANYTHING I CAN DO...
WE APPRECIATE YOUR MEETING WITH US.
ONE YEAR LATER...
TODAY IS THE ANNIVERSARY OF MARY SCHMIDT'S DEATH. ANY WORD FROM HER FAMILY?
NO...
I DID SEND THEM A CONDOLENCE CARD. I STILL FEEL AWFUL ABOUT WHAT HAPPENED.
I'M SURE THEY'RE STILL GRIEVING, ESPECIALLY AROUND THE ANNIVERSARY OF HER DEATH.
DID YOU EVER HEAR FROM THEIR LAWYER?
SHAKE SHAKE
NO, NOTHING.
IT WASN'T SO LONG AGO...
TOP DOCTOR
MARY, CONGRATULATIONS!
THIS MUST BE BABY DONNA.

Battered Trust is based on a true story shared by Dennis Gingrich, M.D., professor of family and community medicine and humanities, member of the board of directors of the American Academy of Family Practice, and a colleague of mine (KM) at Penn State College of Medicine. Although we have modified several details of the case for the purposes of this comic, the essence of it remains the same: a physician makes a mistake that results in a patient's death, decides to admit his mistake, apologizes to the family, and acts to ensure, inasmuch as possible, that such tragedies never happen again under his watch.

Dr. Gingrich shares this story with students every year in their second-year Medical Ethics and Professionalism course. During a broader discussion of medical mistakes and truth-telling, Dr. Gingrich builds a compelling argument that mistakes in healthcare settings are inevitable. Estimating that a physician makes roughly 25,000 decisions per year—a "conservative estimate," he reckons—he points out that every physician, no matter how earnest, careful, and well-qualified he or she is, will make mistakes. After all, when having to make that many decisions, what are the odds that *anyone* could avoid mistakes altogether? Dr. G., as he is affectionately called by both students and patients, cautions aspiring physicians to reject three myths that persist despite our better knowledge: (1) medical mistakes are uncommon; (2) only bad doctors make mistakes; and (3) "I will never make a mistake."

Medical errors occur for many reasons. Some are individual, as in *Battered Trust*, and others are systemic, attributed to no single person but instead the result of processes and procedures that have gone awry. A helpful way to conceptualize such phenomena is the "Swiss cheese model," in which the slices of cheese are metaphors for barriers against mistakes and, despite everyone's conscientious efforts, the holes in those slices align so that a mistake slips through.

Common medical errors are often related to medication—for example, prescribing or administering the wrong drug, the wrong dose, or a bad combination of drugs. Other problems result from workup errors in diagnosis and imaging studies (e.g., missing a key symptom during the physical exam or misinterpreting a CT scan); failure to act on test results; delaying treatment when earlier interventions might have changed the outcome; inadequate follow-up and monitoring; infections, including those from surgical procedures and those from hospital-acquired bacteria; and overtreatment (e.g., delivering too much oxygen, performing too many blood transfusions). When we consider all the ways that errors can occur, it is indeed no wonder that mistakes are inevitable!

Battered Trust illustrates the fallout from Mary's motor vehicle accident: a rupture of her spleen and Dr. G's failure to see the nurse's note that would have helped him diagnose Mary's condition more accurately. The comic also tackles the question of whether one should admit such mistakes—to whom, when, and under what circumstances—highlighting the fact that truth-telling (or lack thereof) impacts the trust at the very heart of the doctor-patient relationship.

Any serious medical mistake brings anguish to patients and families and to the healthcare provider(s) responsible for the mistake. Understandably, a physician's thinking about how to broach the mistake with the patient and family is fraught with fear—given, for one thing, the specter of lawsuits for medical malpractice. It is important to note, however, that research indicates disclosure and apology can have favorable effects on medical malpractice litigation and costs (Robbennolt 376). Even if this were not the case, as of June 2019, thirty-nine states and Washington, D.C., have apology laws that prevent apologies from being admissible in court as an admission of any guilt or wrongdoing (Advisory Board). For example, the Benevolent Gesture Medical Professional Liability Act of Pennsylvania (2013 Act 79) *"applies to any benevolent gesture* made prior to the commencement of a medical professional liability action, administrative action, mediation or arbitration by a health care provider or an officer, employee or agent of a health care provider *to a patient or resident* or the patient's or resident's relative or representative *regarding the patient's or resident's discomfort, pain, suffering, injury or death, regardless of the cause,* resulting from any treatment, consultation, care or service or omission of treatment, consultation, care or service provided by the health care provider" (PA General Assembly; emphasis mine).

While in the United States individual states determine whether to require reporting of medical errors, the culture as a whole seems to be evolving from one that punishes to one that seeks to understand "what happened"—an apparent trajectory from not admitting mistakes to "owning up" to them. In a twenty-first-century society that increasingly demands transparency, "what people will not tolerate is a cover-up, particularly when it pertains to their own health" (Rubel-Seider 505). Rebecca Rubel-Seider, J.D., argues that patients pursue litigation less because they seek monetary compensation than because they want to hold the hospital accountable for the mistake and to protect future patients against similar outcomes. "When the physician offers an apology," she reasons, "the physician reduces the anger of patients, as well as their families, leaving them less likely to pursue litigation" (505).

So what does an effective apology look like? Michael Woods, M.D., proposes five elements of apology for medical contexts: recognition (understanding that an apology is called for), regret (expressing regret for what the patient and family are going through), responsibility (holding oneself accountable for the outcome, even if it could not have been predicted), remedy (doing what it takes to make it right and explaining to patients and families what's being done to prevent a similar mistake from happening to others), and remaining engaged (being present to patients and families throughout the entire process; not withdrawing logistically or emotionally unless patients prefer that another provider take over their care) (Woods i–ix; Bello 1).

To admit one's own responsibility for a negative outcome is to demonstrate respect for those who have suffered from it. Telling the truth and expressing remorse for the mistake is the ethically appropriate course of action, and entities like risk management teams can provide guidance to the physician or other healthcare professional in such situations. The Medical Care Availability and Reduction of Error Act (MCARE) of 2002, which is utilized by states that require reporting of medical errors, outlines guidelines for both verbal and written disclosure—the former to occur "as soon as practical after the unanticipated outcome" and the latter within seven days.

Ultimately, admitting and apologizing for mistakes can help the patient and provider recover and can restore trust in the doctor-patient relationship.

Questions for Further Reflection

1. Consider the delicate balance, as shown in *Battered Trust*, between a physician's "working in" a patient who needs to be seen and the limits on the physician's time and attention.
2. Where does blaming occur in this comic? In each instance, determine how blaming might—and might not—be justified.
3. To what extent do good intentions affect one's response to oversights and other errors in medical judgment?
4. Ponder how you might admit responsibility for a "human error" that had tragic consequences. In your scenario, what might you gain and what might you lose by telling the truth? What factor(s) might tip the scales and lead you to tell the truth—or not?
5. Consider Ms. Kanaan's advice as a representative from risk management. If you were a patient or family member in this scenario, how would a physician's apology impact your future actions and attitudes toward the medical profession? For you, what would a satisfactory apology need to include?
6. Given the history, both distant and recent, between Dr. G. and the Schmidt family, do you believe Donna and Bob would continue medical care with Dr. G. if they had been his patients too?

Note

We thank Dr. Dennis Gingrich for giving us permission to use this story as the basis for *Battered Trust* and to reference his annual lecture on medical mistakes and truth-telling.

Related Readings

Advisory Board. "Do 'Apology Laws' Work?" 17 June 2019, https://www.advisory.com /en/daily-briefing/2019/06/17/apology -laws.

Bello, Mark M. "Malpractice Trial of James Woods' Brother (Michael): The Power of Apology in Litigation." *The Legal Examiner*, 7 December 2009, pp. 1–3.

Gawande, Atul. "When Doctors Make Mistakes." *Complications*, Picador, 2002, pp. 47–74.

Hilfiker, David. "Facing Our Mistakes." *The Social Medicine Reader*, edited by Gail E. Henderson et al., Duke UP, 1997, pp. 287–92.

Kohn, Linda T., Janet M. Corrigan, and Molla S. Donaldson. *To Err Is Human: Building a Safer Health System*. National Academy Press, 2000.

Lazare, Aaron. *On Apology*. Oxford UP, 2005.

PA General Assembly. 2013 Act 79. https://www.legis.state.pa.us/cfdocs/legis /li/uconsCheck.cfm?yr=2013&sessInd =0&act=79, accessed 31 January 2021.

Robbennolt, Jennifer K. "Apologies and Medical Error." *Clinical Orthopaedics and Related Research*, vol. 467, 2009, pp. 376–82.

Rubel-Seider, Rebecca. "Full Disclosure: An Alternative to Litigation." *Santa Clara Law Review*, vol. 48, 1 January 2008, pp. 473–506.

Woods, Michael. *Healing Words: The Power of Apology in Medicine*. 2nd ed., Joint Commission Resources, 2014.

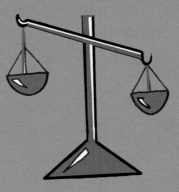

Chapter 7

Surrogate Decision-Making and Advance Care Planning

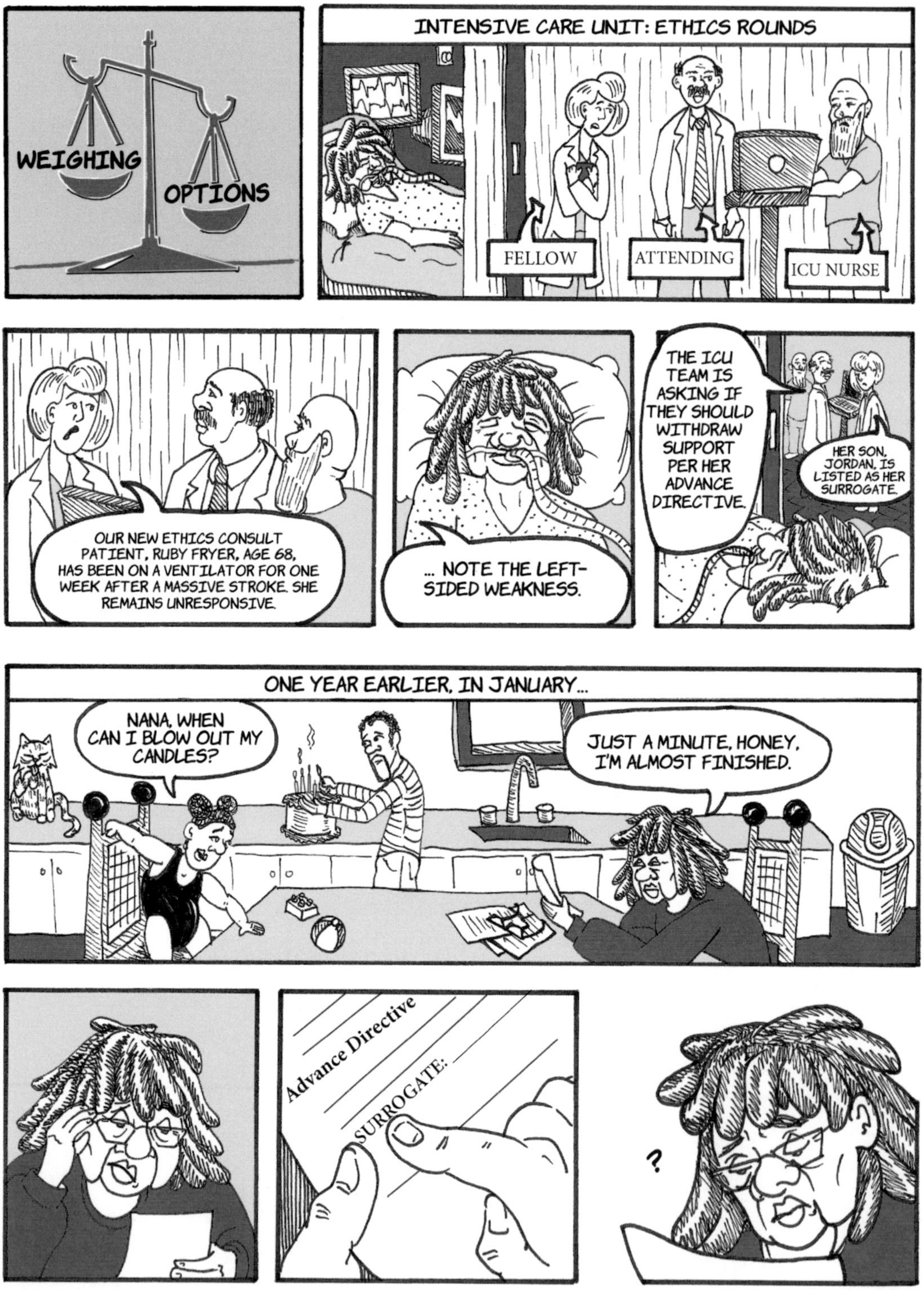
WEIGHING
OPTIONS
INTENSIVE CARE UNIT: ETHICS ROUNDS
FELLOW
ATTENDING
ICU NURSE
OUR NEW ETHICS CONSULT PATIENT, RUBY FRYER, AGE 68, HAS BEEN ON A VENTILATOR FOR ONE WEEK AFTER A MASSIVE STROKE. SHE REMAINS UNRESPONSIVE.
... NOTE THE LEFT-SIDED WEAKNESS.
THE ICU TEAM IS ASKING IF THEY SHOULD WITHDRAW SUPPORT PER HER ADVANCE DIRECTIVE.
HER SON, JORDAN, IS LISTED AS HER SURROGATE.
ONE YEAR EARLIER, IN JANUARY...
NANA, WHEN CAN I BLOW OUT MY CANDLES?
JUST A MINUTE, HONEY, I'M ALMOST FINISHED.
Advance Directive
SURROGATE:
?

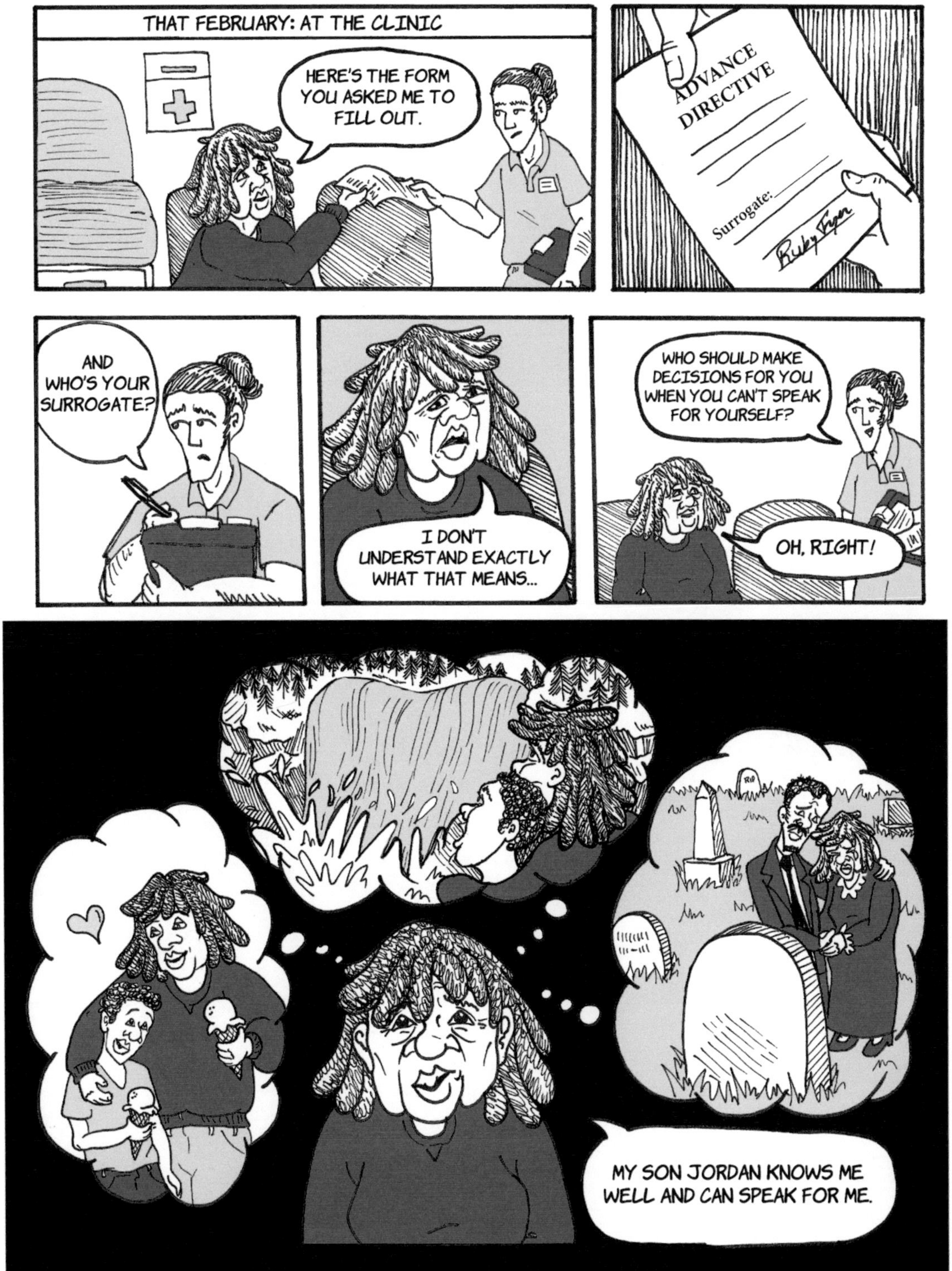
THAT FEBRUARY: AT THE CLINIC
HERE'S THE FORM YOU ASKED ME TO FILL OUT.
ADVANCE DIRECTIVE
Surrogate:
AND WHO'S YOUR SURROGATE?
I DON'T UNDERSTAND EXACTLY WHAT THAT MEANS...
WHO SHOULD MAKE DECISIONS FOR YOU WHEN YOU CAN'T SPEAK FOR YOURSELF?
OH, RIGHT!
MY SON JORDAN KNOWS ME WELL AND CAN SPEAK FOR ME.

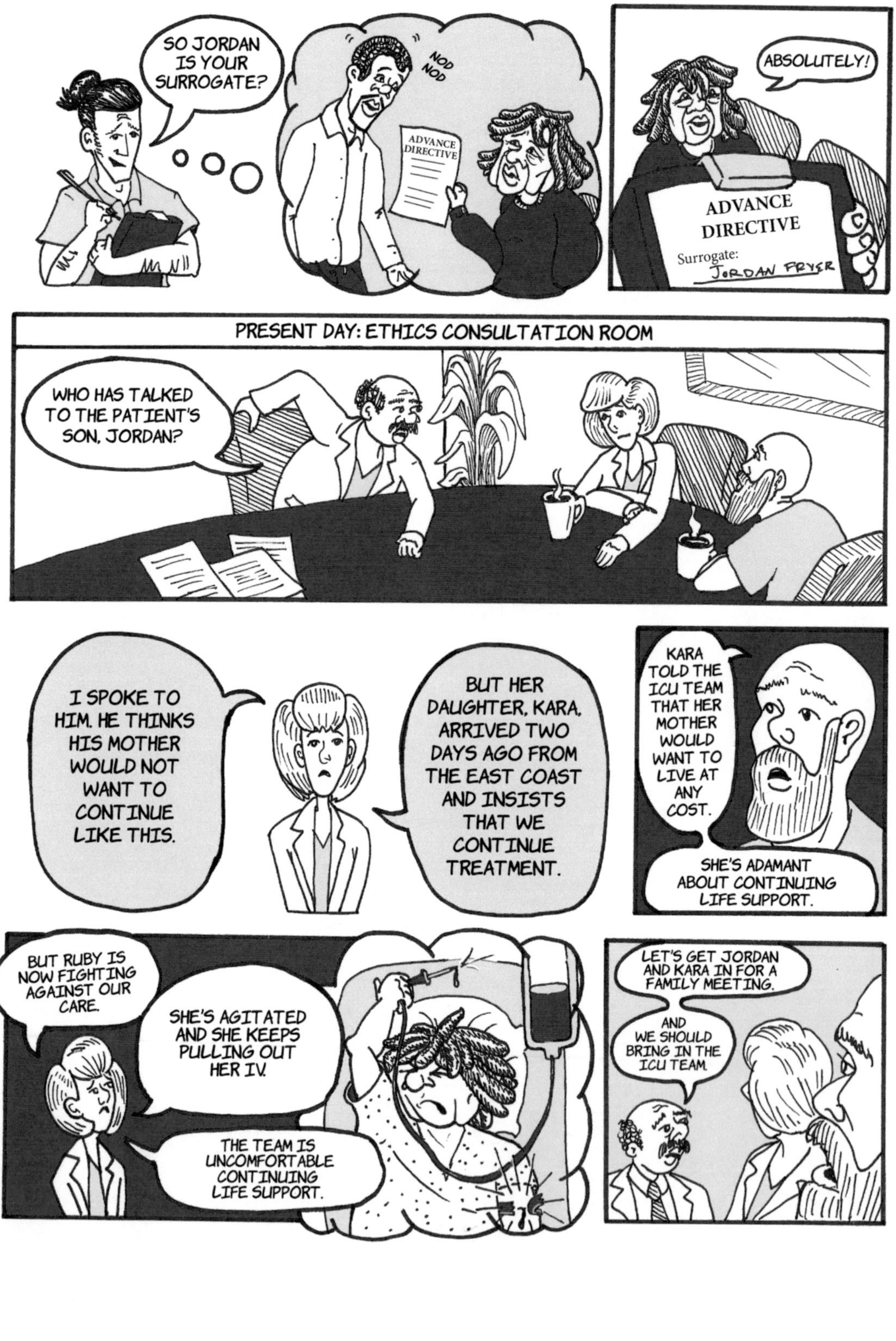
SO JORDAN IS YOUR SURROGATE?
NOD NOD
ADVANCE DIRECTIVE
ABSOLUTELY!
ADVANCE DIRECTIVE
Surrogate: JORDAN FRYER
PRESENT DAY: ETHICS CONSULTATION ROOM
WHO HAS TALKED TO THE PATIENT'S SON, JORDAN?
I SPOKE TO HIM. HE THINKS HIS MOTHER WOULD NOT WANT TO CONTINUE LIKE THIS.
BUT HER DAUGHTER, KARA, ARRIVED TWO DAYS AGO FROM THE EAST COAST AND INSISTS THAT WE CONTINUE TREATMENT.
KARA TOLD THE ICU TEAM THAT HER MOTHER WOULD WANT TO LIVE AT ANY COST.
SHE'S ADAMANT ABOUT CONTINUING LIFE SUPPORT.
BUT RUBY IS NOW FIGHTING AGAINST OUR CARE.
SHE'S AGITATED AND SHE KEEPS PULLING OUT HER IV.
THE TEAM IS UNCOMFORTABLE CONTINUING LIFE SUPPORT.
LET'S GET JORDAN AND KARA IN FOR A FAMILY MEETING.
AND WE SHOULD BRING IN THE ICU TEAM.

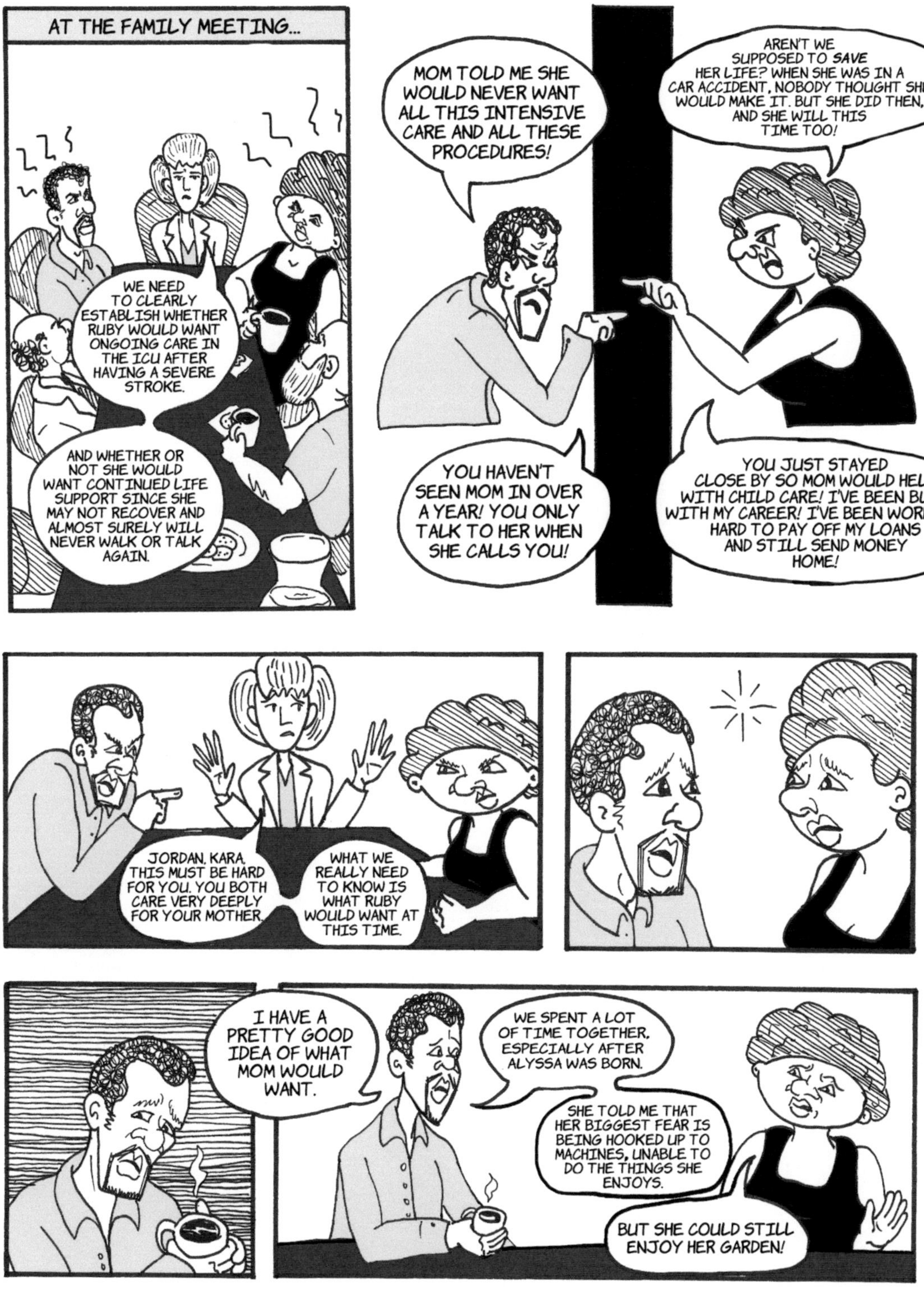
AT THE FAMILY MEETING...
WE NEED TO CLEARLY ESTABLISH WHETHER RUBY WOULD WANT ONGOING CARE IN THE ICU AFTER HAVING A SEVERE STROKE.
AND WHETHER OR NOT SHE WOULD WANT CONTINUED LIFE SUPPORT SINCE SHE MAY NOT RECOVER AND ALMOST SURELY WILL NEVER WALK OR TALK AGAIN.
MOM TOLD ME SHE WOULD NEVER WANT ALL THIS INTENSIVE CARE AND ALL THESE PROCEDURES!
AREN'T WE SUPPOSED TO SAVE HER LIFE? WHEN SHE WAS IN A CAR ACCIDENT, NOBODY THOUGHT SHE WOULD MAKE IT. BUT SHE DID THEN, AND SHE WILL THIS TIME TOO!
YOU HAVEN'T SEEN MOM IN OVER A YEAR! YOU ONLY TALK TO HER WHEN SHE CALLS YOU!
YOU JUST STAYED CLOSE BY SO MOM WOULD HELP WITH CHILD CARE! I'VE BEEN BUSY WITH MY CAREER! I'VE BEEN WORKING HARD TO PAY OFF MY LOANS AND STILL SEND MONEY HOME!
JORDAN, KARA. THIS MUST BE HARD FOR YOU. YOU BOTH CARE VERY DEEPLY FOR YOUR MOTHER.
WHAT WE REALLY NEED TO KNOW IS WHAT RUBY WOULD WANT AT THIS TIME.
I HAVE A PRETTY GOOD IDEA OF WHAT MOM WOULD WANT.
WE SPENT A LOT OF TIME TOGETHER, ESPECIALLY AFTER ALYSSA WAS BORN.
SHE TOLD ME THAT HER BIGGEST FEAR IS BEING HOOKED UP TO MACHINES, UNABLE TO DO THE THINGS SHE ENJOYS.
BUT SHE COULD STILL ENJOY HER GARDEN!

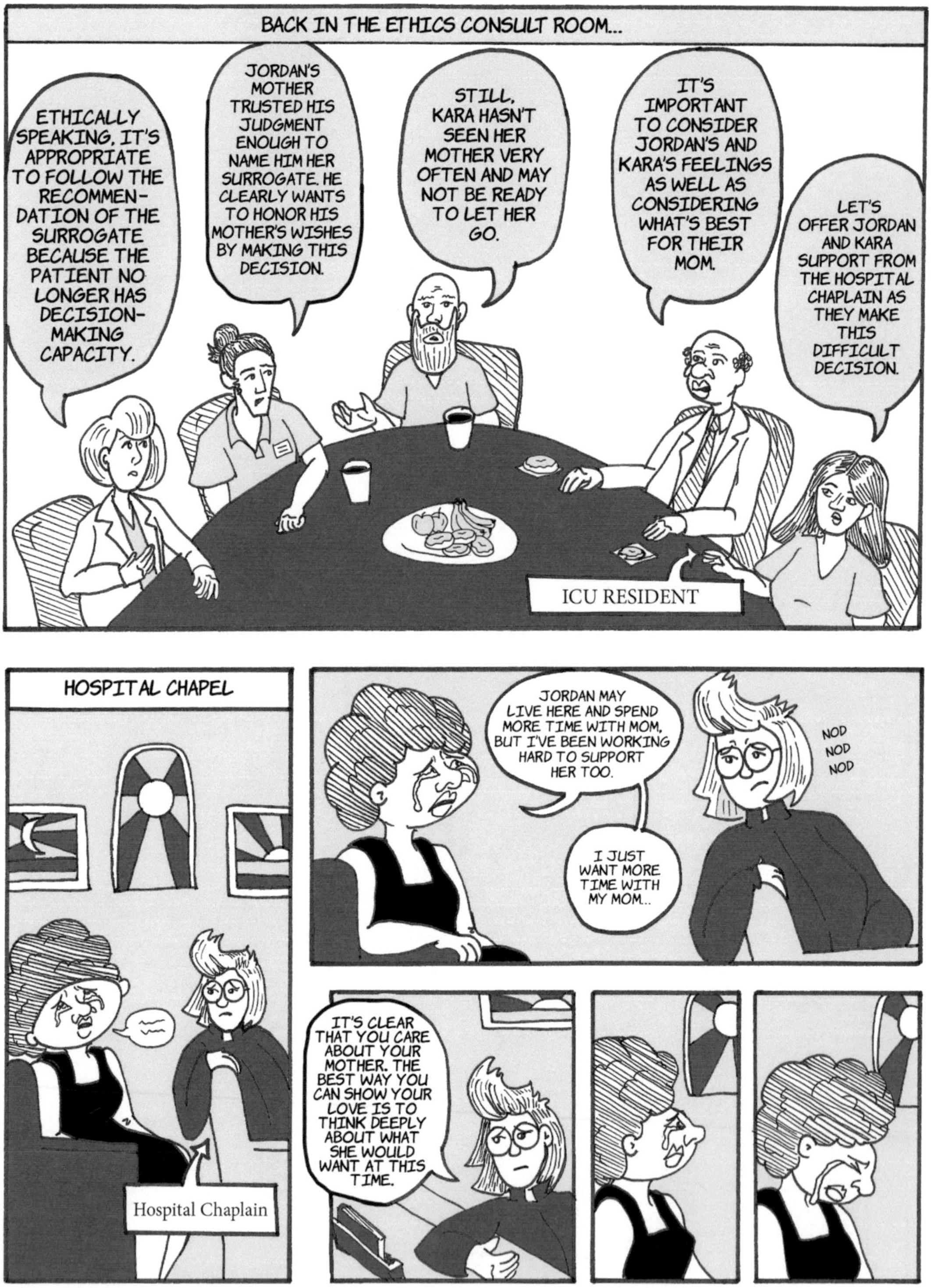
BACK IN THE ETHICS CONSULT ROOM...
ETHICALLY SPEAKING, IT'S APPROPRIATE TO FOLLOW THE RECOMMENDATION OF THE SURROGATE BECAUSE THE PATIENT NO LONGER HAS DECISION-MAKING CAPACITY.
JORDAN'S MOTHER TRUSTED HIS JUDGMENT ENOUGH TO NAME HIM HER SURROGATE. HE CLEARLY WANTS TO HONOR HIS MOTHER'S WISHES BY MAKING THIS DECISION.
STILL, KARA HASN'T SEEN HER MOTHER VERY OFTEN AND MAY NOT BE READY TO LET HER GO.
IT'S IMPORTANT TO CONSIDER JORDAN'S AND KARA'S FEELINGS AS WELL AS CONSIDERING WHAT'S BEST FOR THEIR MOM.
LET'S OFFER JORDAN AND KARA SUPPORT FROM THE HOSPITAL CHAPLAIN AS THEY MAKE THIS DIFFICULT DECISION.
ICU RESIDENT
HOSPITAL CHAPEL
Hospital Chaplain
JORDAN MAY LIVE HERE AND SPEND MORE TIME WITH MOM, BUT I'VE BEEN WORKING HARD TO SUPPORT HER TOO.
I JUST WANT MORE TIME WITH MY MOM...
NOD
NOD
NOD
IT'S CLEAR THAT YOU CARE ABOUT YOUR MOTHER. THE BEST WAY YOU CAN SHOW YOUR LOVE IS TO THINK DEEPLY ABOUT WHAT SHE WOULD WANT AT THIS TIME.

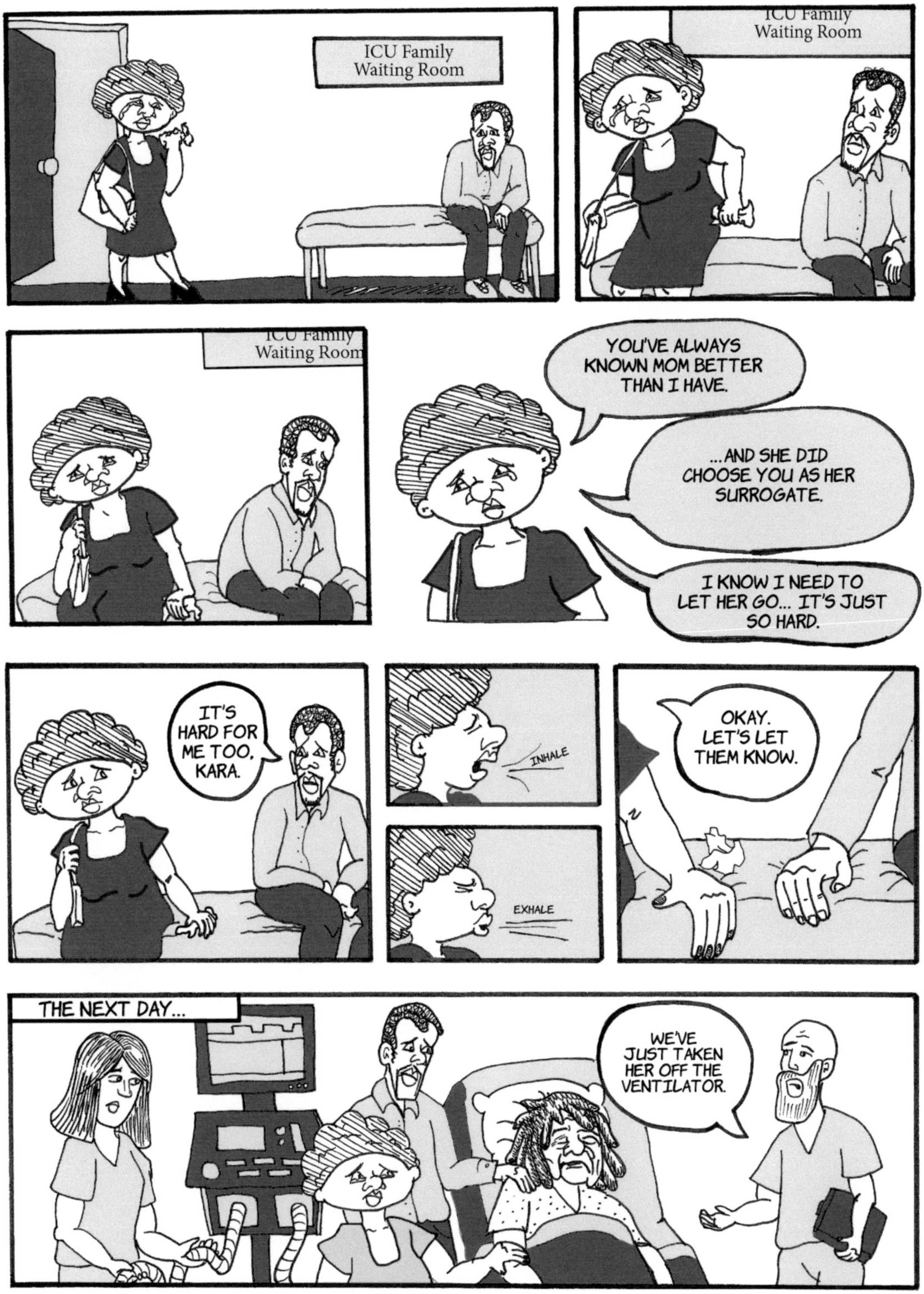
ICU Family Waiting Room
ICU Family Waiting Room
ICU Family Waiting Room
YOU'VE ALWAYS KNOWN MOM BETTER THAN I HAVE.
...AND SHE DID CHOOSE YOU AS HER SURROGATE.
I KNOW I NEED TO LET HER GO... IT'S JUST SO HARD.
IT'S HARD FOR ME TOO, KARA.
INHALE
EXHALE
OKAY. LET'S LET THEM KNOW.
THE NEXT DAY...
WE'VE JUST TAKEN HER OFF THE VENTILATOR.

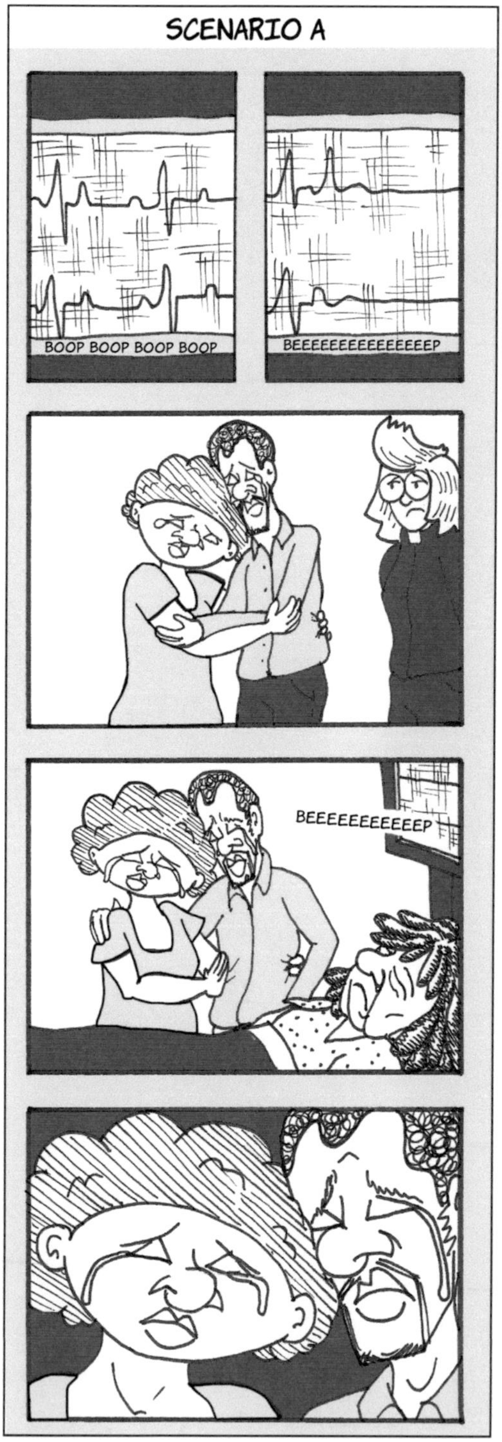
SCENARIO A
BOOP BOOP BOOP BOOP
BEEEEEEEEEEEEEEEP
BEEEEEEEEEEEP

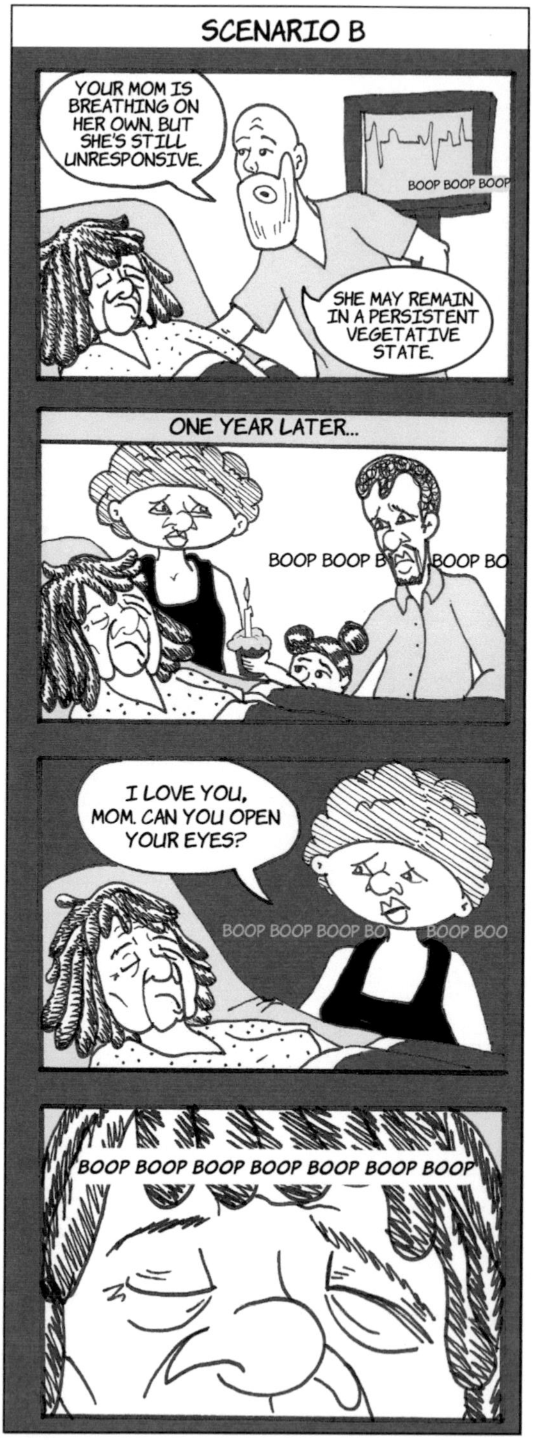
SCENARIO B
YOUR MOM IS BREATHING ON HER OWN. BUT SHE'S STILL UNRESPONSIVE.
BOOP BOOP BOOP
SHE MAY REMAIN IN A PERSISTENT VEGETATIVE STATE.
ONE YEAR LATER...
BOOP BOOP B
BOOP BO
I LOVE YOU, MOM. CAN YOU OPEN YOUR EYES?
BOOP BOOP BOOP BO
BOOP BOO
BOOP BOOP BOOP BOOP BOOP BOOP BOOP

This comic depicts a situation that most families would dread: having to make life-and-death decisions for a person they love when that person cannot communicate a preference. *Weighing Options* addresses the broad topic of advance care planning (ACP), and a key aspect of that process is choosing a surrogate decision-maker who can speak on behalf of the patient when she can no longer make or communicate decisions about her own medical care. ACP can help ensure that a person's wishes are followed in end-of-life decision-making.

Many terms are used in the context of ACP, and they often overlap. The umbrella term "advance care planning" encompasses various forms of advance directives (AD), which are formal documents that specify a person's wishes. Living wills are the most common form of AD. Here, the patient identifies specific preferences for the kind of interventions she would want and not want at the end of her life—whether she would or would not want tube feeding or mechanical ventilation, for instance, as Ruby experiences. Sometimes living wills do not specify decisions for particular situations, perhaps because the patient has not imagined those situations in great detail and therefore has not articulated explicit wishes for each contingency. This is when a named surrogate decision-maker, who knows the patient's preferences well, can speak for the patient.

A surrogate decision-maker (also known simply as a "surrogate" or "proxy") is appointed by a person/patient as part of creating a healthcare power of attorney (HPOA), a legal document that is sometimes also known as durable power of attorney for healthcare (DPAHC). The HPOA speaks on behalf of the person when she cannot speak for herself. If a living will is unclear or does not address a particular situation, the surrogate can step in and speak for the patient, based on the concept of "substituted judgment"—that is, representing the wishes that patient would herself likely have. To apply substituted judgment most effectively, the surrogate will ideally have knowledge not only of the patient's wishes and goals for end-of-life care but also of her core values. This knowledge is helpful because the surrogate can extrapolate from a given situation about which the patient *has* commented to other similar situations about which she has not explicitly spoken. If for some reason the surrogate is unable to represent the patient's wishes via substituted judgment, the surrogate would then apply the "best interests" standard, which involves making a determination of what would be best for the patient, given the competing benefits and burdens of a particular medical intervention—for example, whether to continue kidney dialysis in the context of a persistent vegetative state. This standard for decision-making is notably more subjective than the substituted judgment standard.

Ultimately, the objective of surrogate decision-making is to represent and hence respect the patient's wishes, and for this reason, decisions made by the surrogate take precedence over choices that are, or might be, made by members of the family who are not the patient's surrogate. As such, it is helpful for the surrogate to be named early in the patient's care and for him or her to come to appointments with the patient, especially appointments with the patient's primary care physician. This enables the physician to assess the surrogate's willingness and ability to carry out the role and, equally important, to have met the surrogate before a medical crisis requires the surrogate's presence. Because these joint meetings are collaborative, they can provide greater clarity for the surrogate and therefore presumably help him or her make difficult decisions with less anguish when the time comes.

Advance care planning can be confusing and daunting for patients and families. Consequently, it is important for healthcare providers to encourage patients and families to prioritize these kinds of discussions and to help them navigate the process.

Questions for Further Reflection

1. Where in the comic do you see implicit references to substituted judgment and best interests? How do these concepts play out differently depending on the "stakeholders," including the family members and various members of the healthcare team who are present?

2. What is the role of the chaplain in this comic, and how does she contribute to the care of the patient?

3. As authors of the comic, we deliberately chose to depict reconciliation between Jordan and Kara, and their respective perspectives, in order to encourage thinking beyond the decision itself. Consider the impact of Jordan and Kara's decision on themselves and on their mother in Scenario A and then in Scenario B. Such reconciliation among persons and perspectives is not always the case. How might Ruby's story have played out if her children had continued to disagree about what was best for her? What constitutes a "good" outcome?

4. Consider "moral distress" as it appears in *Weighing Options* and *Critical Space*. How do the differences in clinical situations impact the moral distress of the family members and healthcare providers?

5. Alongside *Weighing Options*, consider the case of Terri Schiavo in the 1990s and early 2000s.

Related Readings

Annas, George J. "'Culture of Life' Politics at the Bedside—The Case of Terri Schiavo." *New England Journal of Medicine*, vol. 352, no. 16, 21 April 2005, pp. 1710–15.

Balaban, Richard B. "A Physician's Guide to Talking About End-of-Life Care." *Journal of General Internal Medicine*, vol. 15, March 2000, pp. 195–200.

Sudore, Rebecca L., and Terri R. Fried. "Redefining the 'Planning' in Advance Care Planning: Preparing for End-of-Life Decision Making." *Annals of Internal Medicine*, vol. 153, no. 4, 17 August 2010, pp. 256–61.

Winkenwerder, Jr., William. "Ethical Dilemmas for House Staff Physicians: The Care of Critically Ill and Dying Patients." *The Social Medicine Reader*, edited by Gail E. Henderson et al., Duke UP, 1997, pp. 230–35.

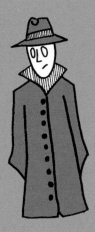

Chapter 8

Futility

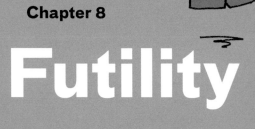

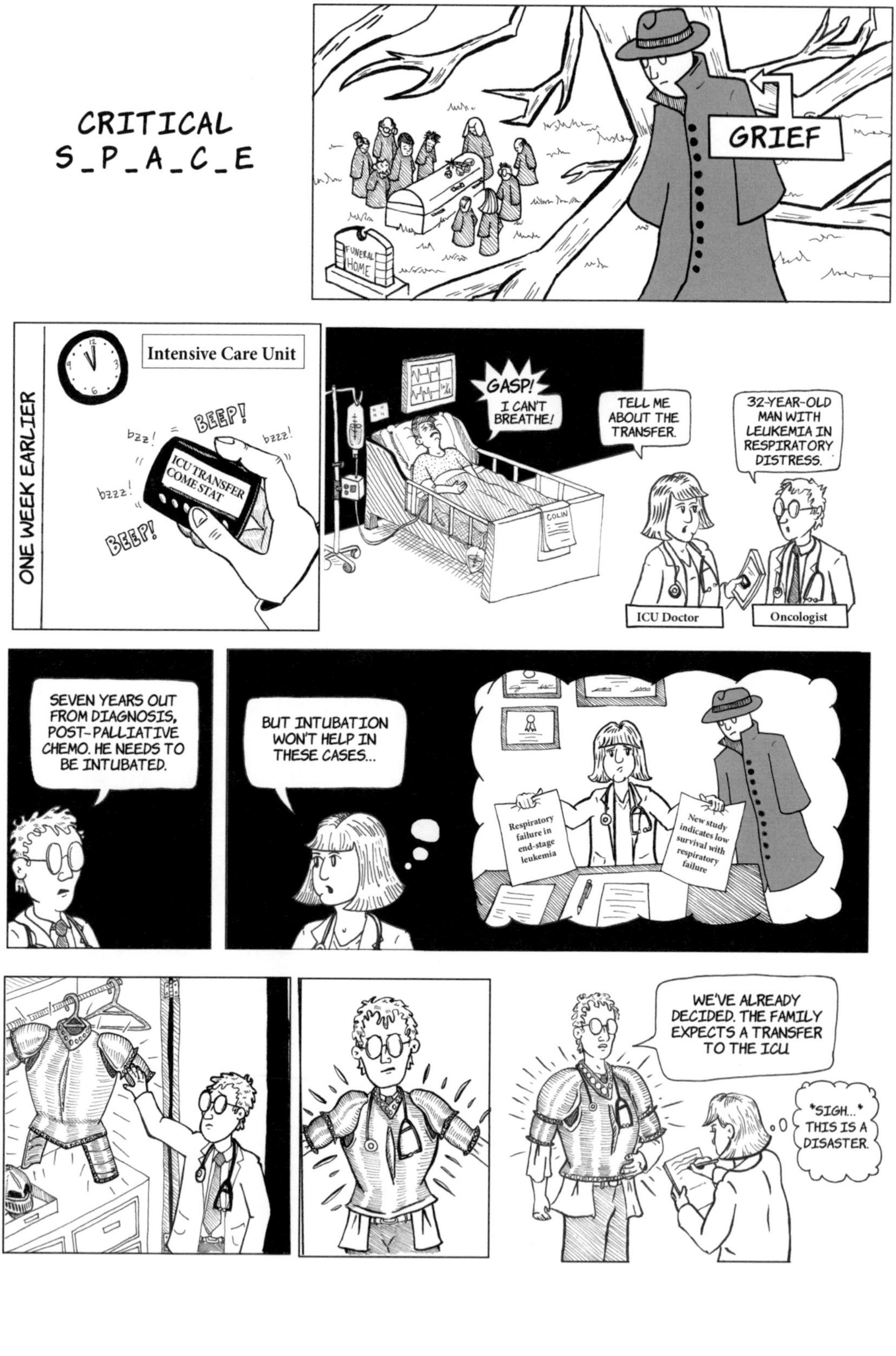
CRITICAL
S_P_A_C_E
FUNERAL HOME
GRIEF
ONE WEEK EARLIER
Intensive Care Unit
BEEP!
bzz!
bzzz!
bzzz!
ICU TRANSFER COME STAT
BEEP!
GASP! I CAN'T BREATHE!
COLIN
TELL ME ABOUT THE TRANSFER.
32-YEAR-OLD MAN WITH LEUKEMIA IN RESPIRATORY DISTRESS.
ICU Doctor
Oncologist
SEVEN YEARS OUT FROM DIAGNOSIS, POST-PALLIATIVE CHEMO. HE NEEDS TO BE INTUBATED.
BUT INTUBATION WON'T HELP IN THESE CASES...
Respiratory failure in end-stage leukemia
New study indicates low survival with respiratory failure
WE'VE ALREADY DECIDED. THE FAMILY EXPECTS A TRANSFER TO THE ICU.
SIGH... THIS IS A DISASTER.

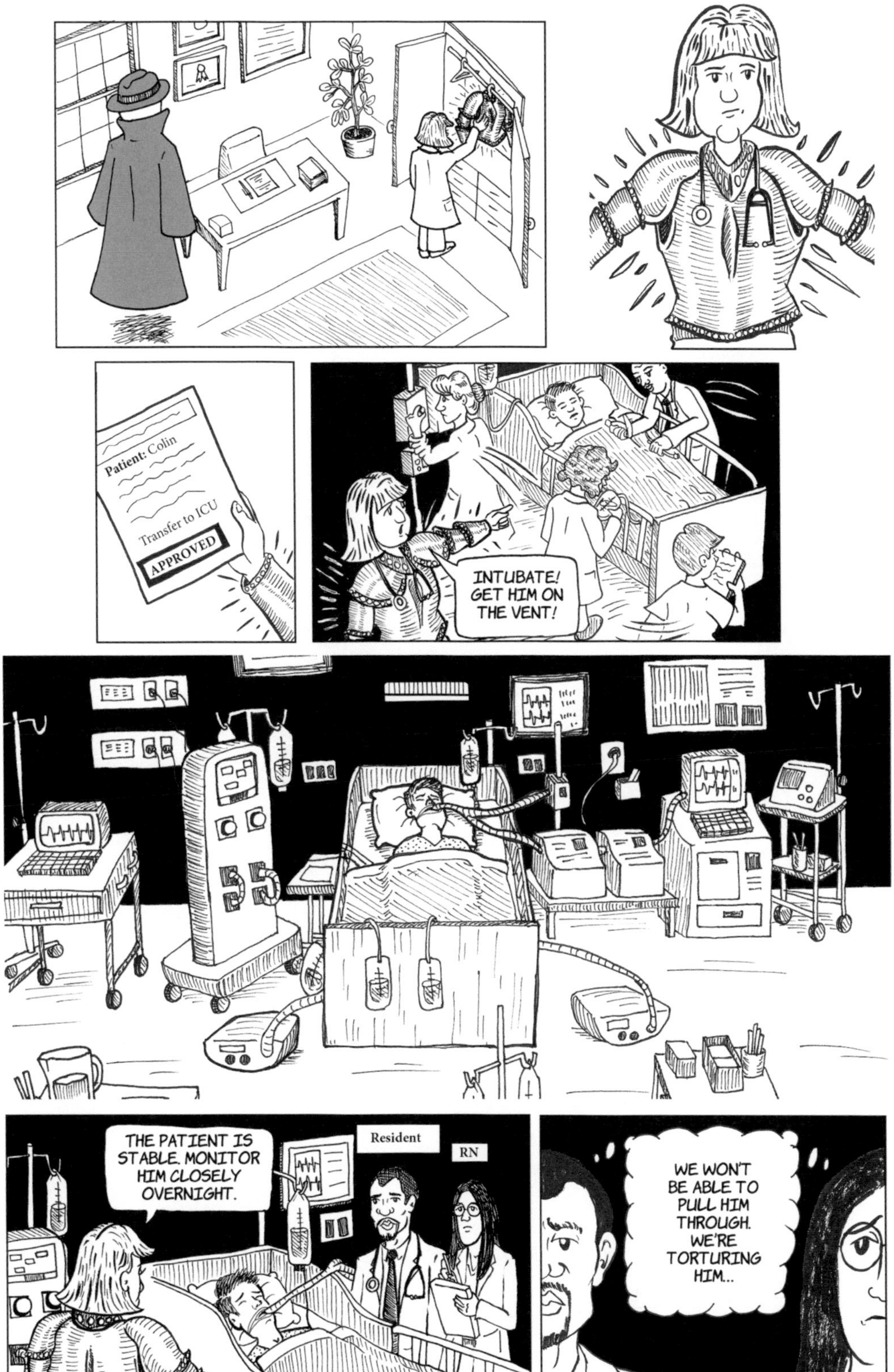
Patient: Colin
Transfer to ICU
APPROVED
INTUBATE! GET HIM ON THE VENT!
THE PATIENT IS STABLE. MONITOR HIM CLOSELY OVERNIGHT.
Resident
RN
WE WON'T BE ABLE TO PULL HIM THROUGH. WE'RE TORTURING HIM...

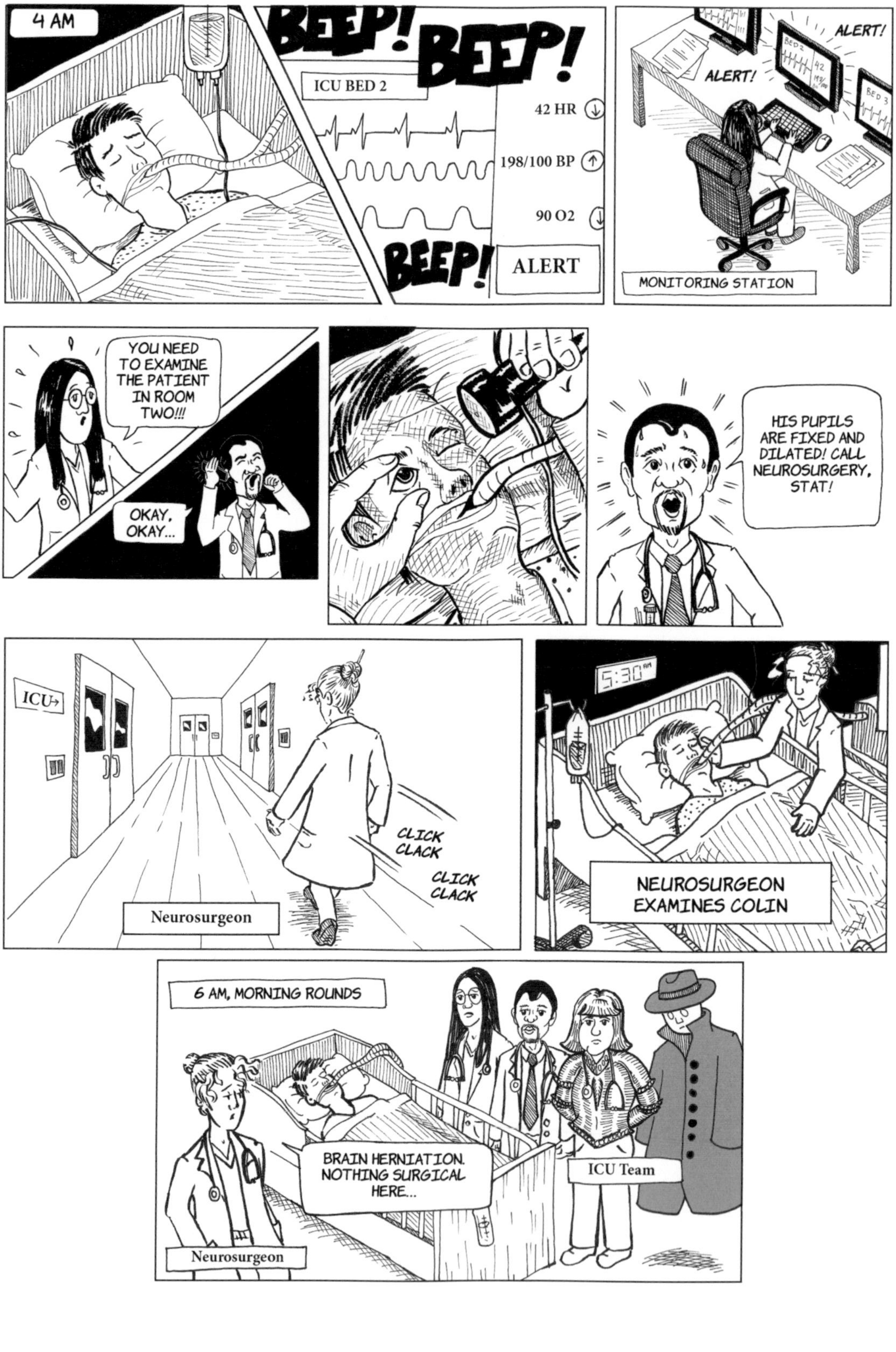
4 AM
BEEP! BEEP!
ICU BED 2
42 HR
198/100 BP
90 O2
BEEP!
ALERT
ALERT!
ALERT!
MONITORING STATION
YOU NEED TO EXAMINE THE PATIENT IN ROOM TWO!!!
OKAY, OKAY...
HIS PUPILS ARE FIXED AND DILATED! CALL NEUROSURGERY, STAT!
ICU
CLICK CLACK
CLICK CLACK
Neurosurgeon
5:30
NEUROSURGEON EXAMINES COLIN
6 AM, MORNING ROUNDS
BRAIN HERNIATION. NOTHING SURGICAL HERE...
ICU Team
Neurosurgeon

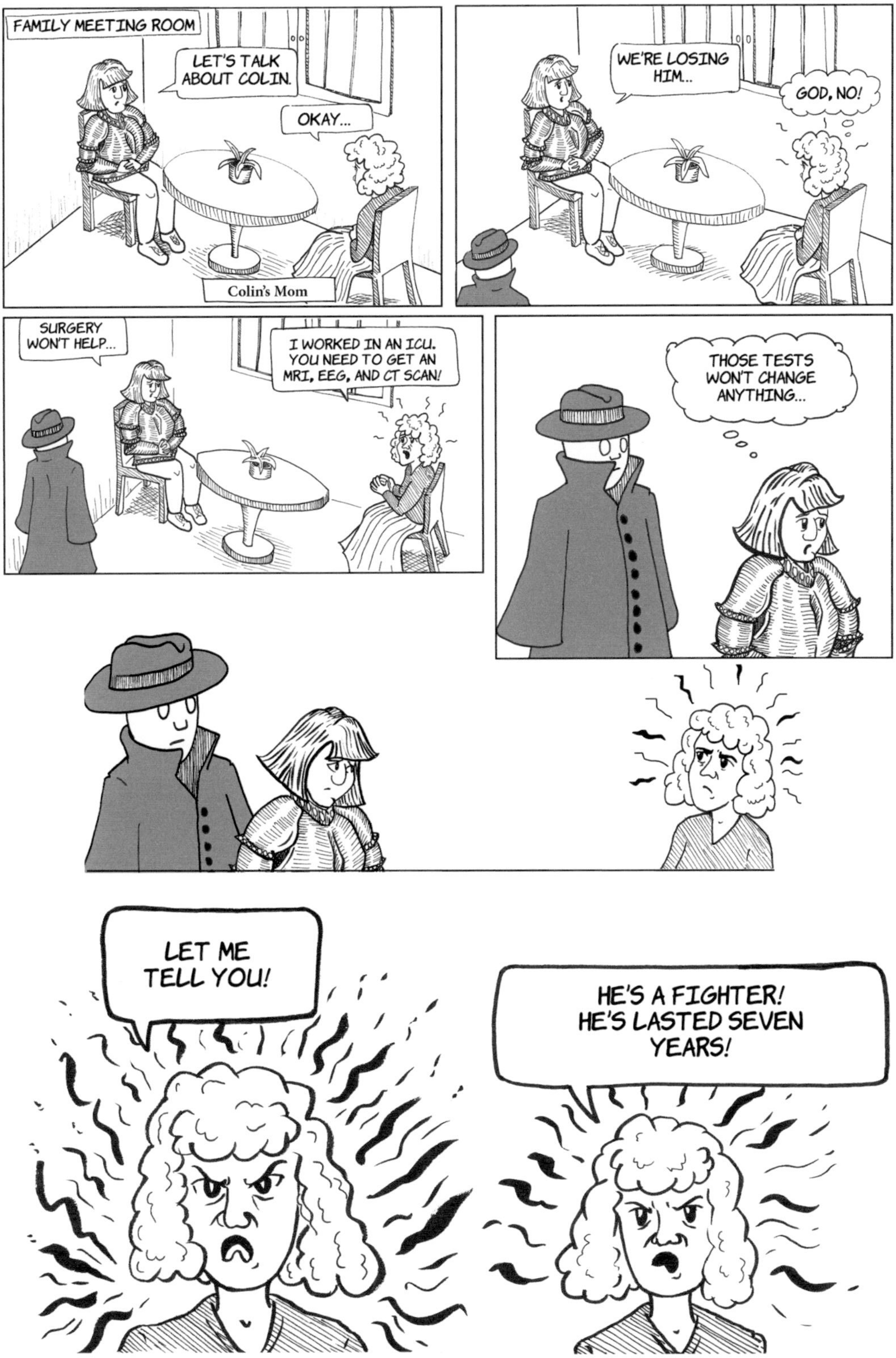
FAMILY MEETING ROOM
LET'S TALK ABOUT COLIN.
OKAY...
Colin's Mom
WE'RE LOSING HIM..
GOD, NO!
SURGERY WON'T HELP...
I WORKED IN AN ICU. YOU NEED TO GET AN MRI, EEG, AND CT SCAN!
THOSE TESTS WON'T CHANGE ANYTHING...
LET ME TELL YOU!
HE'S A FIGHTER! HE'S LASTED SEVEN YEARS!

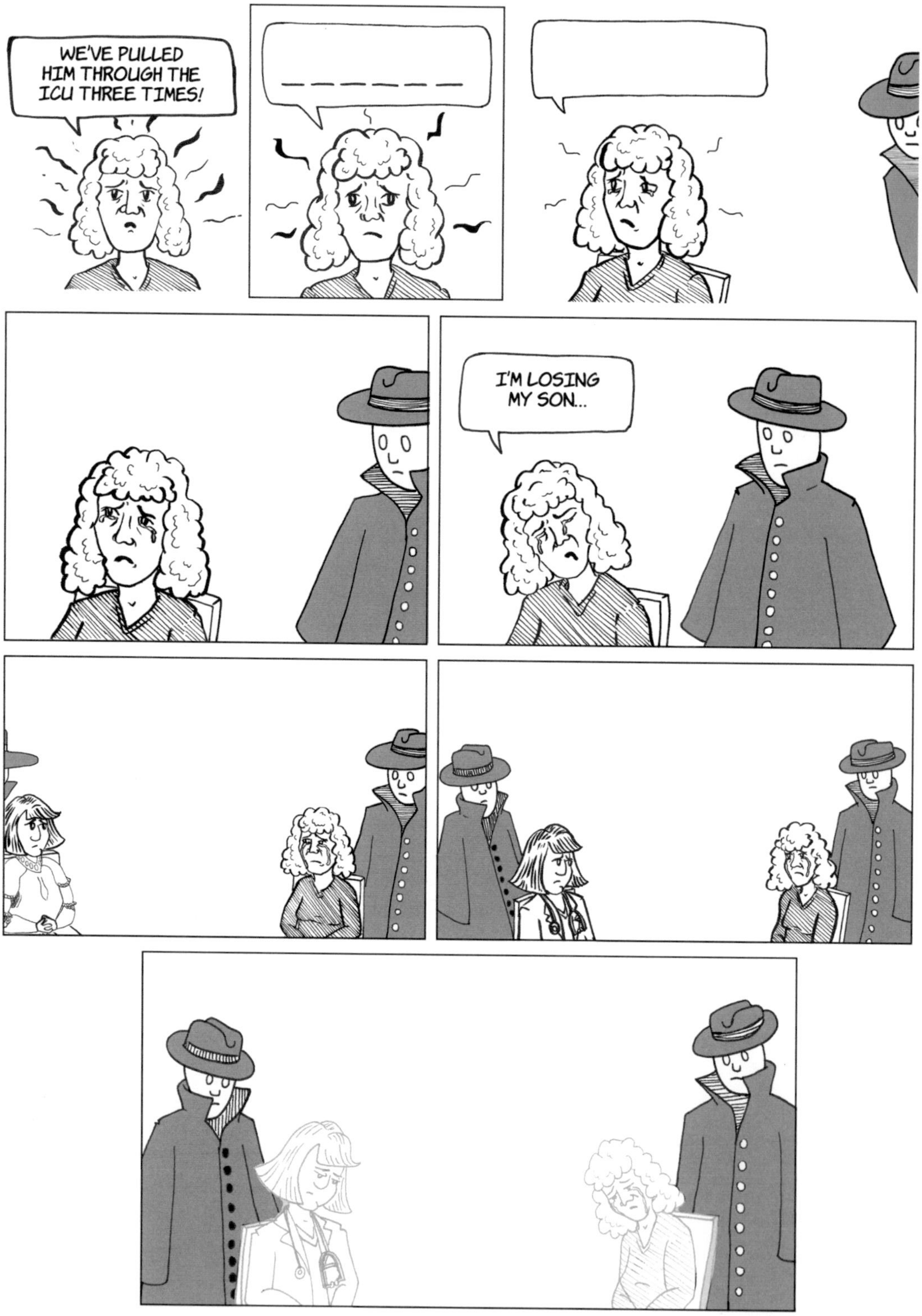
WE'VE PULLED HIM THROUGH THE ICU THREE TIMES!
I'M LOSING MY SON...

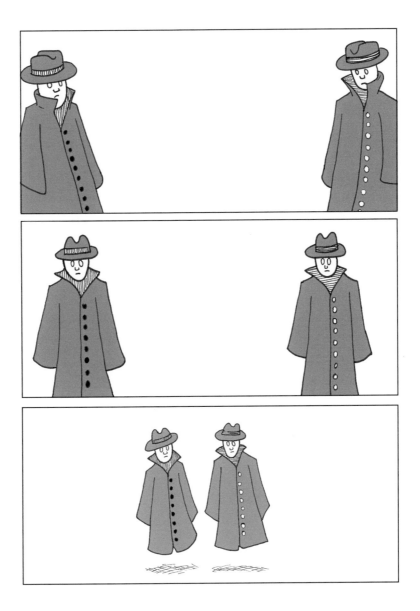

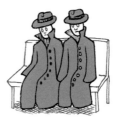

Discussion

Critical Space raises a number of issues relevant to end-of-life care, including the often misunderstood concept of futility, a situation in which medical treatment will almost certainly fail to save a person's life. Colin's blood cancer has advanced to the point that his medical team has given him "palliative" chemotherapy. Because meaningful recovery for Colin is no longer possible, chemotherapy is meant only to alleviate symptoms like pain and dyspnea (shortness of breath). Ironically, his worsening respiratory failure may be a result of the palliative chemotherapy that he has received—a predicament that reveals the delicate balance between the benefits and risks of medical interventions.

The intensive care unit (ICU) doctor recognizes how things stand with Colin. Acknowledging that people in his condition who develop serious breathing complications rarely survive, she understands that intubation (inserting a breathing tube) will not likely accomplish the goal of prolonging life. We aren't told why the oncologist recommends that Colin be transferred to the ICU, but it is almost surely in part because the family has asked for the next level of medical care: "Family expects transfer to the ICU," the oncologist insists. The wheels are now set in motion for Colin to be intubated and placed on a ventilator (breathing machine), which raises the ethical question of whether complying with the family's wishes would be futile.

Healthcare providers often invoke the concept of futility when they believe an intervention is not worthwhile, but doing so risks muddying already confusing waters. Medical ethicist and pediatrician Benjamin Levi, M.D., Ph.D., offers a helpful way to think of futility: consider whether an intervention is *possible* (fact-based; will it work?) versus whether an intervention is *worthwhile* (values-based; is it beneficial?). Levi poses the example of hauling water out of a flooded basement using a thimble. It can be done, but it's probably not a good use of time or resources.

Griffin Trotter, M.D., Ph.D., also a medical ethicist and an emergency medicine physician, points out that for an intervention to be considered futile, three conditions must be met: (1) there must be a goal, (2) there must be an action aimed at achieving the goal, and (3) there must be virtual certainty that the action will fail to achieve the goal. Though parties in the debate may disagree about the wisdom or value of pursuing the goal, this is conceptually distinct from futility, which addresses whether the proposed intervention can accomplish the goal. Quite simply, whether something is worthwhile is different from whether it is indeed "futile."

In *Critical Space*, Colin's mother recognizes that further tests can be obtained to evaluate his clinical situation and that it might be possible to keep her son alive for a period of time. She insists on more studies even though, as a former ICU nurse, she knows *intellectually* that the tests won't change anything. This time the issue is personal for her, so logic doesn't prevail—at least not immediately. However, she comes to realize that the use of technology will not "bring him back"; technology will not restore her son's consciousness and previous quality of life. He will not recover.

Providers' reasons for discontinuing treatment can extend beyond the narrow construct of futility; their concerns can be medical or moral. When death is inevitable and imminent, the burdens of treatment typically outweigh the benefits for the patient, and the provider must strike a balance between the principles of beneficence (doing good for the patient) and nonmaleficence (avoiding harm to the patient). At other times, an issue of resource allocation may be at play—for example, as seen during the 2020 COVID-19 pandemic, when there were concerns about shortages of intensive care beds and ventilators.

When providers sense that they are doing more harm than good with their medical interventions, they can despair. In *Critical Space*, the resident and registered nurse think, "We're torturing him," and the intensive care doctor calls the situation a "disaster." Such experiences can negatively impact healthcare providers' ability to provide compassionate care, because moral distress can lead to burnout, distracted focus, and emotional distancing. Recognizing this danger, the American Medical Association has determined that physicians are not ethically obligated to deliver care that, in their best professional judgment, will have no reasonable chance of benefiting their patients: "Respecting patient autonomy does not mean that patients should receive specific interventions simply because they (or their surrogates) request them."

Questions for Further Reflection

1. Why is grief personified in two different but similar figures? When does Grief appear and why?
2. What does the armor symbolize? Who wears armor (and who does not)? How is that important in the story? When do physicians put on armor and why? What causes armor to disappear?
3. In what ways does this comic explore various "critical spaces"? What is critical here? What kinds of spaces exist?
4. Contemplate the last five panels. What's going on here? What's the nature of the relationship between the two figures of Grief? Why are they depicted sitting side by side at the end?
5. Alongside *Critical Space*, consider the cases of Karen Quinlan, Nancy Cruzan, and Helga Wanglie.

Note

We thank Dr. Benjamin Levi for giving us permission to cite examples and illustrations from his annual lecture on futility at Penn State College of Medicine.

Related Readings

American Medical Association. "Medically Ineffective Interventions: Code of Medical Ethics Opinion 5.5." http://www .ama-assn.org/delivering-care/ethics /medically-ineffective-interventions, accessed 7 May 2021.

Miles, Steven H. "Informed Demand for 'Non-Beneficial' Medical Treatment." *The Social Medicine Reader*, edited by Gail E.

Henderson et al., Duke UP, 1997, pp. 403–6.

Trotter, Griffin. "The Concept of Futility." *Cambridge Quarterly of Healthcare Ethics*, vol. 8, 1999, pp. 527–37.